THE
PLANT-BASED
BOOST

*Nutrition Solutions for Athletes
and Exercise Enthusiasts*

Melissa Halas MA, RDN, CDE

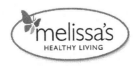

Paperback ISBN: 978-1-7339692-2-2
Hardcover ISBN: 978-1-7339692-3-9
Ebook ISBN: 978-1-7339692-4-6

Senior Editor
Claire Haft, MS, RDN

Cover and Interior Layout
Streetlight Graphics, LLC

The information provided in this book is for general informational purposes only.

No representations or warranties are expressed or implied about the information, products, services, or related graphics contained in this book for any purpose.

To my parents, family, and relatives who never waiver in their love and support, thank you. I'm so blessed to have you in my life.

Table of Contents

Chart and Table Index

There is a range of variability allowed for nutrition labeling. Nutritional values are often rounded up or down and can differ based on nutrition analysis software. There are variables within a species. For example, there are several types of white beans. Also, food inherently has unique nutrient values due to many factors, including soil type, fortification, and testing method.

Author Acknowledgement

Thank you to the reviewers, athletes, and sports dietitians who helped fine-tune and evaluate this book's content to make it come together over the past several years. Special gratitude goes to my senior editor, Claire Haft, whose kindness and patience was very evident through the many tedious editing sessions. I appreciate your unwavering encouragement and ability to access research articles in seconds. You got me to the finish line!

A special thank you to my colleagues who have inspired me during my twenty-year journey in nutrition and dietetics, and to my students who I love and appreciate so much. Another big thanks to my clients, who ensure that I stay up to date on a variety of nutrition topics and the latest food trends! All of you provide me with a constant source of inspiration.

About the Author

Melissa Halas, MA, RDN, CDE is a Registered Dietitian Nutritionist, Certified Diabetes Educator, and wellness expert. She has 20 years of diverse experience in nutrition education, nutrition counseling, curriculum development, clinical care, clinical trials, media, and writing. Melissa is the current media representative for the California Academy of Nutrition and Dietetics, the parent nutrition expert for the People.com online magazine, and a past panel expert on Childhood Obesity for TedMed.

Through her company, Melissa's Healthy Living, she provides nutrition counseling to help clients of all ages – including athletes – reach their best genetic potential. Melissa believes balanced nutrition contributes to positive spiritual, physical, and mental health. For 18 years she taught functional foods, sports nutrition and other courses, which developed her love for more than one specialty while offering a rewarding and diverse career in nutrition. Melissa is also the founder of SuperKids Nutrition, a mega site and premier source for kids and family nutrition, and is the creator of the Super Crew®, a group of multi-cultural characters who get their powers from healthy plant-based foods and motivate young children to develop healthy eating habits from an early age.

Getting Started

Y OU'VE MADE IT! YOU'VE TAKEN your first step towards a more plant-based lifestyle! And no, this doesn't mean you have to say goodbye to meat forever. You're about to embark on a journey to understand the ins and outs of what "plant-based" truly means, how to fuel properly for your exercise, and all that this eating pattern can do for your overall health and your athletic performance. Let's dive in!

A carbohydrate and protein-rich diet are essential for optimal performance and recovery, enabling athletes and exercise enthusiasts to work harder, faster, and longer. Whether you're an omnivore (all foods), pesco-vegetarian (fish + dairy + eggs), vegetarian (eggs +/- dairy), or vegan (100% plants), plant-based proteins can improve your health, optimize your athletic performance, and help you feel and look great while decreasing age-related diseases.

There are three macronutrients, carbohydrate, protein, and fat, that provide our bodies with energy. These macronutrients may or may not be accompanied by vitamins, minerals, fiber, and plant compounds called phytonutrients—also known as phytochemicals—in our food.

First, what exactly are plant-based proteins? They are plant-based foods that contain notable amounts of protein. They also naturally contain carbohydrates (including fiber), and some of them offer a source of healthy fat. After reading this, you'll master the plant-based eating basics and understand how the specific nutrition profiles of these foods can help you reach your performance goals and improve your long-term health!

We'll start out explaining the ins and outs of protein, then dive into the role carbohydrates play in energy production, and review the many benefits of protein-rich carbohydrates. We'll discuss the benefits of heart-healthy fats while debunking some common fat myths. To top this all off, we'll give you some insight into phytonutrients and take a closer look at supplements and performance enhancing foods.

How to Read This Book

Every athlete or exercise enthusiast has unique goals. There are many variables at play when developing a fitness and nutrition plan – gender, age, body composition, genetics and more. Utilize the resources provided in this book to come up with your individualized solution to optimize your performance, fitness level, and health. All athletes can benefit from boosting plant-based foods for their health and our planet.

The term athlete is defined as a person who is proficient in sports or other forms of physical exercise.

The term exercise enthusiast is defined in this book as a person who exercises regularly in their choice of fitness as a hobby or for good health.

Don't sell yourself short – anyone who is working out at least 6-8 hours a week, including at least two days of muscle-strengthening activities that are moderate or high-intensity, can consider themselves athletes. Each person's fitness and physique goals are unique based on their athletic pursuits, individual and family health history, and overall wellness goals. Most sports are classified by intensity and duration, but for this book, we broke it down further to help you focus on key areas of nutrition that apply specifically to you. Regardless of your sport, all athletes and exercise enthusiasts benefit from phytochemicals and the right types and amounts of carbohydrates, protein, and fats in addition to the focus areas below. Keep in mind that some sports can overlap depending on your training plans, such as strength and endurance. It's difficult to pigeonhole one sport or exercise to a specific category.

1. **Endurance sports** – distance running, distance cycling, mountain biking, distance swimming, triathlons (longer than sprint distance), marathons, full-day events
   - carb loading
   - nutrition during exercise
   - hydration
   - increasing specific foods to minimize oxidative stress or improve blood flow
   - recovery nutrition: pairing carbohydrate and protein

2. **High-intensity, short-duration sports requiring strength and power** – gymnastics, sprint cycling, sprinting, hurdles, track sports, swimming, football, martial arts, fencing, CrossFit, track events, wrestling
   - macronutrient (carbohydrates, protein, fat) basics
   - calculating carbohydrate and protein needs
   - recovery nutrition: pairing carbohydrate and protein

3. **Team/individual sports, and stop-and-go sports using all energy systems** – soccer, lacrosse, tennis, basketball, rowing, hockey, rugby, football, rock climbing
   - carbohydrate and fluid intake to maximize event performance
   - recovery nutrition: pairing carbohydrate and protein

4. **Physique sports** – bodybuilding, jockeys, gymnasts, dancers, boxers
   - may apply the protein section of this book more diligently calculating grams of protein per day, especially for body composition goals
   - macronutrient basics and balancing meals for overall health and longevity

5. **Exercise enthusiasts** – indoor cycling, Pilates, yogis, hikers, general gym members
   - macronutrient basics for weight management
   - may focus on grams of protein per kilogram per day to increase muscle mass while training
   - healthy fats and phytonutrients for an anti-inflammatory diet due to a specific family health history

6. **Activity requiring motor control, coordination, reaction time** – golf, Pilates, etc.
   - general information on protein, carbohydrate, fat, and hydration

No matter what type of athlete you are, or the intensity of your training or exercise program, this book will help you understand the benefits of plant-based proteins and plant-based foods for your unique goals. Throughout the book, the term athlete is all-encompassing. At certain points, there will be distinct differences noted between elite athletes, competitive athletes and exercise enthusiasts. However, the nutritional needs of athletes and exercise enthusiasts are similar. So, if you're not sure where you fall within a specific nutrition recommendation, see what works best for you with trial and error. Individuals in each category of activity can benefit from boosting plant-based eating, and this eating pattern can successfully support performance at all levels of competition!

 There are some topics that are a bit "technical" that really focus on nutrition science. We've marked these with this atom symbol. Feel free to skip over these sections and come back to them later when your brain is in full power mode for a deeper look at the science.

Book Objectives

Understand that your overall nutrition needs and the availability of your energy resources can be influenced by many factors, some of which include:

- gender
- age
- body weight and body composition
- overall nutritional status
- diet composition
- lifestyle patterns (meal timing, sleep, stress)
- environment (i.e., temperature)
- type and level of training
- eating strategy around exercise
- drugs and/or supplements
- sport or event

Note that this book will not be covering specific considerations for health conditions that could impact recommendations and strategies during exercise. This includes but is not limited to athletes with specific medical diagnosis such as diabetes, gastrointestinal diagnoses, or a compromised immune system. Since nutritional guidance for such conditions is out of the scope of this book, we highly recommend working with a Registered Dietitian Nutritionist.

The companion recipe book, *The Plant-Based Boost Cookbook, 100+ Recipes for Athletes and Exercise Enthusiasts* will show you how to meet your nutritional needs in a simple and delicious way.

How a Plant-Based Diet Can Work for You

As you saw with the exercise classifications, exercise encompasses a wide range of sports and activities that rely on different training routines, nutrition approaches, and many other factors. You've likely chosen a sport or exercise program that is enjoyable and makes you feel great. Staying active and boosting those "feel good" endorphins are at the core of good health. Finding the balance of doing enough activity, while also making sure you don't do too much, should be the first step to ensure good health and to keep that enjoyment alive.

Exercise routines that meet the exercise guidelines for Americans (per the

U.S. Department of Health and Human Services) have been shown to stimulate the immune system and improve overall health (even more reason to keep your heart pumping and your body moving!).[1] However, prolonged, intense exercise or overtraining can compromise the immune system. What's considered overtraining varies between individuals. Signs of overtraining could include excessive fatigue, poor performance, increased respiratory infection, and viruses, or in women, amenorrhea.[2,3] These are, of course, all things we want to avoid, and are partly in our control.

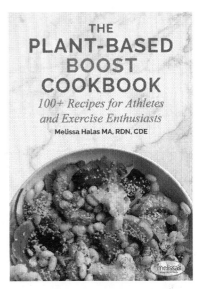

THE
PLANT-BASED BOOST COOKBOOK
100+ Recipes for Athletes and Exercise Enthusiasts
Melissa Halas MA, RDN, CDE

melissas

Additionally, exercise can result in tissue damage as part of the muscular adaptation to exercise. This is a normal function of exercise and shouldn't be confused with muscle injury. During tissue damage and the resulting tissue repair, inflammation results as a natural healing mechanism. This inflammation is a vital step to muscle growth and repair. However, long term or chronic inflammation can compromise athletic performance and overall health.

So How Does Boosting Plant-Based Foods Come to the Rescue?

Research has clearly established that vegetarian diets are associated with improved health outcomes. Diets like the Mediterranean and DASH (Dietary Approaches to Stop Hypertension) diet that have a high percentage of plant-based foods are associated with lower incidence of inflammation.[4,5] A recent comprehensive meta-analysis showed a significant protective effect of a vegetarian diet, decreasing mortality from ischemic heart disease by 25% and decreasing cancer risk by 8%. Vegan diets offered additional protection, showing a 15% decreased risk from cancer.[6] This shows that boosting plant-based foods is good for overall health and longevity.

We know that carbohydrates still get top billing for high-performance athletes, and inadequate carbohydrates can lead to performance losses and negative impact on training capacity.[7,8] Eating adequate carbohydrate also helps sustain muscle energy reserves in athletes and exercise enthusiasts. Because plant-based proteins and a plant-based diet are higher in carbohydrate, they help foster effective glycogen storage.

Overall, vegetarian diets offer these advantages:

- reduced risk of morbidity and mortality from ischemic heart disease, metabolic syndrome, and lower levels of total cholesterol, LDL, and triglycerides[6,11]
- lower blood pressure
- reduced risk of cancer
- decreased risk of developing type 2 diabetes
- higher glycogen stores
- often associated with reduced body fat and leaner body composition[9]
- contain higher intake of plant compounds and antioxidants which: [6,10,11]
    - help lower inflammation as noted by lower levels of C-reactive protein
    - decrease oxidative stress, improving immunity
    - improve arterial flexibility
    - improve blood flow
- may have an alkaline effect compared to a non-vegetarian diet[10]
    - theoretically, increasing plant-based foods may increase serum alkalinity, which is correlated with an increase in physical performance
- higher intake of vitamin C, vitamin E, and beta-carotene, in comparison to omnivore diets, which can further reduce exercise-induced oxidative stress[11]
- lower levels of uric acid – high levels of uric acids are linked to gout, arthritis and other chronic diseases

By boosting plant-based foods you are moving closer to the benefits. Plant-based food intake varies based on individual lifestyle approach and taste preferences. Therefore, the level of health benefit varies in degree as well. This is why it's key to have a flexible approach that works for you! Food should be enjoyed just as you enjoy your active lifestyle.

Food Memories and Their Influence

Think back to a time when you went to a restaurant or friend or family's home that offered a specific type of cuisine that you tried and disliked. What are your feelings toward that food today? It's theorized that our brain creates simulations around the thought of food – how it may taste and what we'll experience. These simulations are most often influenced by previous times we tried a similar food, which constructs an idea in our minds of what the new experience will be. If our experience was negative, these constructs may inhibit us from trying a new dish. When considering a new plant-based food, start by focusing on the flavor, look, and feel. This focus should replace the pattern of retrieving a past experience. In addition to our memories of food, the names of a dish may influence us as well. Food sales have demonstrated that people can attach negative feelings towards food labeled meat-free, vegan, vegetarian or that uses healthy language.[12] The way foods are listed and named have influence over what we purchase or order. For example, the name, "Cuban black bean soup," versus "vegan black bean soup" creates a different perception. The Cuban black bean soup has been shown to be significantly more appealing.[12] Pay attention to your own biases and how they shape, limit or enhance your openness to boosting plant-based foods in your diet.

Keep the Outdoors Happy for Your Outdoor Activity

The outdoors are easy to take for granted since they're there every day for us without question. They offer a place for a morning run, bike ride, hike, or other enjoyable activity in the fresh air. Our food choices may seem far from impacting the air we breathe, but they have more of an impact than we may realize. Small changes add up over time and can positively impact the air you breathe and even the terrain you climb during interval training or a nice relaxing run. Making a choice to adopt a more plant-based diet can be a simple step that you do for your long-term health while decreasing the environmental impact. It was found that a "25% reduction in meat consumption and transition to vegetarian eating patterns would minimize the impact of agricultural land expansion on ecosystems, biodiversity, and carbon dioxide emissions."[13] Even switching from eating beef on a regular basis to primarily fish and poultry can make a big difference.[13]

Living the green life is healthier for you AND it's better for the planet. This green mentality is really just about focusing on more local products, organic goods, fresh fruits and vegetables, and foods high in nutrients but low in added sugars and chemical preservatives. Other environmental benefits to being greener include reducing the use of pesticides and herbicides released into the environment, promoting ocean health by supporting sustainable fishing practices, and reducing carbon emissions. Lucky for us, the foods that are best for our health typically have a more positive impact on the environment!

Fruits, vegetables, whole grains, legumes, lentils, nuts, and seeds all come from the ground and require much less energy to produce than meats. Eating these plant-based foods helps reduce the production of greenhouse gases. Per the United Nations, 14-18% of global greenhouse gases are from livestock.[14] To add to this, about 80% of agricultural land is utilized for livestock's grain consumption. To meet the world's protein needs we are going to see a big shift towards plant-based proteins. Considering the majority of athletes and exercise enthusiasts spend much of their time outdoors, and would like to preserve their outdoor environment, who could be better suited to lead the way to promote plant-based foods?

You can use carbon dioxide equivalents as a measure of how much your food choices impact the environment. For example, a black bean bowl has 254 grams of carbon dioxide equivalent emission (co2-eq) per bowl versus a bowl of beef chili which has 2,449 grams of co2-eq.[15] The beef chili has nearly ten times more emissions!

Per the World Resource Institute, beef is resource intensive to produce, requiring 20 times more land and emitting 20 times more green gas emissions per gram of edible protein than common plant proteins, such as beans, peas, and lentils.[16] Even more astounding is that beef alone accounts for 36% of our food-supply-related emissions.[17]

This chart by the World Resources Institute shows a simple comparison of the environmental impact of different foods, in addition to the typical cost of those foods. Overall, the plant-based foods are better for the environment and are friendlier to your wallet.

Organic Food Choices

Eating organic is a personal choice, just like all food choices. You can decrease your pesticide intake and promote environmental health by including organic foods in your diet when possible. You might already know that eating plant-based foods benefits your health by lowering your risk of chronic diseases. The most important part of a healthy diet is getting enough fruits, vegetables, whole grain, beans, nuts, and seeds. Pesticides or not, including a variety of plant-based foods in your daily routine should be priority number one!

Seasonal Eating and Food Waste

Seasonal eating also makes a positive impact on the planet and can save

PROTEIN SCORECARD

What you put on your plate has a large impact on the environment. Research by WRI and its partners shows that meat and dairy are generally more resource-intensive to produce than plant-based foods, increasing pressure on land, water and the climate. Small dietary shifts—such as switching from beef to pork, or poultry to beans—can significantly reduce agricultural resource use and greenhouse gas (GHG) emissions. Use this scorecard to lower your diet's impacts in a way that works for you.

Read more at **wri.org/shiftingdiets**   join the conversation **#ShiftingDiets**

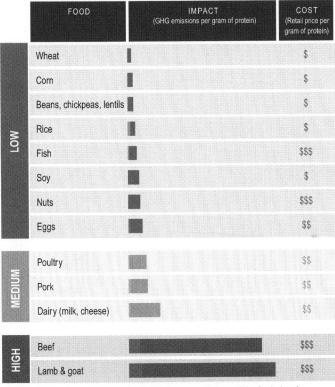

	FOOD	IMPACT (GHG emissions per gram of protein)	COST (Retail price per gram of protein)
LOW	Wheat		$
	Corn		$
	Beans, chickpeas, lentils		$
	Rice		$
	Fish		$$$
	Soy		$
	Nuts		$$$
	Eggs		$$
MEDIUM	Poultry		$$
	Pork		$$
	Dairy (milk, cheese)		$$
HIGH	Beef		$$$
	Lamb & goat		$$$

Lighter shade shows emissions from agricultural production, darker shade shows emissions from land-use change.

How Much Protein Do You Need?

The average daily adult protein requirement is **56g** for a man and **46g** for a woman but many people consume much more than they need.

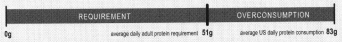

REQUIREMENT	OVERCONSUMPTION
0g average daily adult protein requirement **51g**	average US daily protein consumption **83g**

Sources: GlobAgri-WRR model developed by CIRAD, Princeton University, INRA, and WRI (GHG data); USDA and BLS (2016) (US retail price data).   *Notes:* see www.wri.org/proteinscorecard.

Source: World Resource Institute[16]

on cash. Seasonal produce has trekked fewer miles to make it to your plate. If you're having trouble figuring out which foods are in season, stop by the farmer's market or take a look at the produce that's on sale in your grocer's produce section.

About 28% of our carbon footprint is due to food loss and waste.[17] Make sure to freeze your leftovers before they expire. These extra portions can come in handy after a long, hard workout when you're too tired to cook - and you'll be helping our planet!

Balance is Key

You likely know how important physical and mental balance is for you. Nutritional balance is just as essential. Finding an enjoyable and healthy approach to nutrition as an athlete or exercise enthusiast is key to your success. It's easy to over-focus on certain aspects of nutrition, such as protein intake, and forget about other important factors that come into play. Eating a balanced diet as an athlete helps you make optimal gains in your training and performance, enhances recovery time, lowers your risk of acute and chronic health issues, and helps you achieve your optimal physique.

Here are common nutritional issues that often present with athletes in nutrition counseling sessions:

- not getting enough carbohydrates or whole grains
- concern about taking in too much fat, which is essential for cushioning
- inadequate fruit, vegetable, fiber, and omega-3 fatty acids (referred to as omega-3s)
- over-focusing on protein intake, while skimping on carbohydrates or fats
- not understanding protein's significant role and that additional protein and calories are needed for muscle gains
- not consuming enough carbohydrates and fat to help protect and preserve muscle as an energy source
- unwanted weight loss or weight gain
- poor hydration
- inadequate electrolyte or carbohydrate intake during training and competition days
- food budget concerns

Melissa Halas MA, RDN, CDE

- lack of meal planning skills
- poor knowledge of key nutrients
- incorrect or unsafe supplementation

NUTRITION TIP

There's more to good nutrition than carbohydrate, protein, fat, vitamins, and minerals. Don't forget water, fiber (a form of carbohydrate that your body can't break down – more on this later), and phytonutrients that are abundantly found in plant-based foods.

Part 1:
PROTEIN - THE MASTER SYNTHESIZER

A PROTEIN-RICH DIET IS ESSENTIAL FOR optimal performance and recovery which all starts with amino acids. Amino acids are the building blocks of protein, and your body links amino acids together to build proteins. The essential amino acids (ones we have to get from our diet) are crucial drivers of muscle-building through muscle protein synthesis. Learning how to get creative with plant-based protein is key to reaching your protein needs in a day. It is possible to entirely meet your needs for physical performance with plant-based proteins, without having to rely on animal protein.[10]

In addition to providing athletes with some essential amino acids and stored energy in the form of carbohydrates, the essential vitamins and minerals in plant-based proteins have the potential to boost athletic performance while reducing the risk of chronic disease and maximizing overall wellbeing. Exercise enthusiasts get the same benefits and can tailor their nutrition to meet their physique and health goals. Plus, plant-based proteins typically cost much less than animal proteins and offer more variety!

Now let's take a closer look at protein and all that it does for your body. You'll no longer have to guess how to evaluate your diet to make sure you're getting a variety of beneficial plant-based proteins.

Protein's Leadership Role

Whether derived from animal or plant sources, protein is the captain for building muscle and driving muscle recovery and contributes to an athlete's overall athletic performance. It is also important for those who want to build or maintain muscle mass and manage weight goals, or for people who are recreationally active. You'll learn why soon.

Just like a championship-winning team, protein can't excel without the support of its teammates! Together with protein, there are the other five key players we mentioned before – carbohydrates, fats, water, vitamins, and minerals. Fiber and phytonutrients are important too. These all work together to help maximize your performance and recovery, and ensure

Melissa Halas MA, RDN, CDE

you are properly fueled for your gym session, practice, training day, game, or next big race.[18,80]

Protein's Tough Responsibilities

Protein is an essential macronutrient with unique roles in the body. Some of protein's many responsibilities are:[20]

- enzyme and hormone synthesis
- formation of organs and cellular structures
- supporting your immune system
- maintenance of fluid balance
- development of transport proteins (including those that carry oxygen through the blood)

You can see that protein plays a crucial role in a variety of processes in our bodies. Under certain circumstances, even though it isn't a preferred or desirable fuel source, protein becomes a vital source of energy for the body during exercise. This happens when carbohydrate stores have been exhausted, after running a marathon or another endurance-type activity, or when an athlete under-consumes carbohydrates. This is why it's key to consume adequate carbohydrates – you want to avoid using protein from your muscle or from the protein you eat as much as possible. It's also important to keep in mind that trying to fuel exercise with protein is not as efficient as with carbohydrates and may accelerate fatigue or decrease your time to exhaustion. This is why dietitians and nutrition scientists always say, "Carbohydrates are good and necessary, especially for fitness!"

Plant-based proteins provide the best of both worlds – giving you amino acids for building muscle and carbohydrates with slowly digested fiber for long-lasting energy to power through your workouts.

It's better to maintain protein within muscle or use it to fulfill all the responsibilities listed above instead of being broken down for energy due to inadequate carbohydrate intake.

Types of Protein

To stay alive you must consume protein! That's why it's considered one of the six essential nutrients. Protein is composed of carbon, oxygen, hydrogen, and nitrogen, and is broken down by the body into amino acids for absorption. Amino acids are considered the building blocks of protein, and they fulfill various vital functions in the body. As you train, your muscles break down to release amino acids for your body to use. The protein you get from your diet must provide sufficient amino acids to repair your muscles and prepare you for continued training at the same high intensity. This is why it can be helpful to track your protein for a few days. Keep in mind that all athletes and exercise enthusiasts require different amounts of protein based on training type, intensity, volume, and individual body composition and performance goals. Before we get into protein specifics for you, let's touch on the basics.

**So now that you know what protein does,
you may be wondering...does the type of protein matter?
Is all protein equal?**

Amino Acids

There are 20 amino acids that are divided into three main categories – essential, nonessential, and conditional. If an amino acid is essential, it must be obtained through the diet. As you can guess, nonessential means the body can make that specific amino acid by itself. The amino acids classified as conditional are ones that the body can synthesize mostly on its own, except in certain circumstances. During times of illness or stress, or if there is a lack of certain resources within the body, you must consume foods that contain those amino acids to meet the body's demand. This is why it's important to eat a wide variety of protein sources throughout the day.

There is an amino acid pool in our body which is constantly turning over protein. Some protein is being synthesized or built up from amino acids, while others are being degraded or broken down into amino acids. Therefore, your body continually has access to all types of amino acids to build muscle (and support all of protein's other roles) and meet your protein needs, when eating a balanced diet.

Here is a list of the essential amino acids. Don't feel like you have to memorize these. It's mostly just to serve as a reference when we talk about some of them throughout the book.[20]

Essential

Histidine	Lysine	Threonine
Isoleucine*	Methionine	Tryptophan
Leucine*	Phenylalanine	Valine*

*Branched-chain amino acid

Animal Protein

Most animal proteins, such as meat, fish, poultry, eggs, milk, cheese, and yogurt, are considered complete proteins because they contain all nine of the essential amino acids needed by the body in sufficient amounts.[20] One ounce of cooked animal protein (like cooked fish or cooked chicken) provides 7 grams of protein. The downside of animal proteins is that many of them contain saturated fat, don't contain fiber, and produce more carbon emissions. As you'll learn throughout this book, this is the opposite of almost all plant-based proteins.

Plant Protein

Plant-based proteins do contain some amino acids; however, most of them lack one or more essential amino acids, and are, therefore, considered incomplete protein sources.[20] This doesn't mean you can't thrive without animal protein; there are many ways to make sure you're getting the right nutrients – even as a vegan!

However, it may take a bit of planning to eat a vegan or vegetarian diet to make sure you're getting the quality and amount of protein required by your body. Successful vegan athletes eat a variety of essential amino acids from different plant-based sources throughout the day and week in order to meet their needs. Decades ago plant-based proteins were paired at meals to make a complete protein. Today we know that the adequacy of plant-based proteins is based on a full day, not just on one meal. Eating a variety of plant-based foods ensures that you are getting all of the essential amino acids you need – each plant protein will contain essential amino acids that another food might not have.

Remember, you don't have to be vegan or vegetarian to get the benefits of plant-based proteins. They can fit into any diet! You can choose what works for your lifestyle. You don't want to miss out on their health benefits, as they contain certain vitamins and minerals, fiber, and phytonutrients not found in animal protein. These nutrients help fight off chronic disease, including osteoarthritis (especially in the knee), type 2 diabetes, heart disease, and many types of cancer.[21-23] Plus, they help with healthy skin, hair, nails, and the immune system.

PLANT POWER

Phytochemicals, also known as phytonutrients, are plant compounds that have endless health benefits. We call them "fight-o-nutrients" because they fight off disease! Make sure you get a variety of these compounds by including a colorful variety of foods throughout the day – each color provides unique phytonutrients to give you an extra boost.

The main food groups we are targeting when we say plant-based proteins are:

- legumes (beans – including soy, peas, lentils, peanuts)
- whole grains
- nuts
- seeds

Keep in mind that while 1 ounce of a protein-rich animal food has approximately 7 grams of protein, the amount of protein in plant foods varies. One ounce is 2 tablespoons. See portion chart below and keep these insights in mind:

- Most vegetables have 2-3 grams of protein per 1 cup, cooked.
- Most grains have 2-3 grams of protein per ½ cup, cooked. We'll provide you with a detailed chart later on.
- Most legumes have around 12-14 grams protein per 1 cup, with lentils having the most.

Serving size examples

- **Woman's fist or baseball** – 1 cup of vegetables or fruit
- **A rounded handful** – extend your hand out, the circle (minus the fingers) is considered about ½ cup cooked or raw veggies, cut fruit, or a piece of fruit – this is a good measure for a snack serving, such as baked tortilla chips or plantain chips
- **Deck of cards or the palm of your hand (minus the fingers)** – a 3-ounce serving of meat, fish or poultry – for example, one chicken breast, quarter-pound hamburger patty, or a medium pork chop

- **Golf ball or large egg** – ¼ cup of dried fruit or nuts
- **Tennis ball** – about 1 cup of pasta or ready-to-eat cereal
- **Computer mouse** – 1 small baked potato
- **Thumb tip** – 1 teaspoon of nut or seed butter

YOUR TURN

Go to your calendar and schedule in a time to track protein intake for two weekdays and one weekend day. Don't worry whether or not you're meeting a requirement - track it to get a sense of your eating patterns now, before you're influenced by what you read in the following pages.

Legumes and pulses

Legumes include soybeans, peanuts, fresh peas, and fresh beans. Pulses are part of the legume family and include beans, lentils, chickpeas, and peas. The term "pulse" refers only to the dry edible seed within the pod. Pulses are rich in protein, fiber (including resistant starch), folate, iron, antioxidants, and lignans and saponins (phytochemicals).[24-27]

Lignans are a group of phytonutrients that may help prevent heart disease and lower inflammation.[28] Saponins are a type of plant compound that may help lower cholesterol, boost immunity, and decrease cancer risks.[29]

Many people are surprised to learn that peanuts are a legume and are not considered a true nut. Here are a few of our favorite legumes:

- black beans
- pinto beans
- kidney beans
- cannellini beans
- garbanzo beans

- black-eyed peas
- green peas
- split peas
- lentils
- peanuts

Soy proteins, followed by legumes, are the plant-based proteins with the highest concentrations of the essential amino acids.

Soy

Soy is an excellent source of plant-based protein and includes foods such as tofu, soymilk, edamame, and more. It is one of the few plant-based proteins that *do* contain all essential amino acids, is low in fat, and high in calcium (when fortified). Some forms are fermented, such as tempeh, which is a great source of probiotics – beneficial bacteria that live in your gut. Unfortunately, soy is often a very polarizing food. There are firm believers on both ends of the spectrum, but we will provide the evidence below to show you the science behind why soy is a beneficial component to a healthy diet.

Breast Cancer

Soy contains phytoestrogens – plant-derived estrogen – and it has been widely misrepresented that eating high amounts of phytoestrogens will heighten the risk of breast cancer. However, in practice, the opposite effect has been shown in specific types of breast cancer. Previously, the research has been limited to Asian cultures that typically consume high soy diets, leading some scientists to hypothesize that these ethnic groups innately process soy differently. Newer research, however, has shown similar results with Caucasian participants, refuting those claims, and further highlighting the potential benefits of consuming soy due to the isoflavone content. Human studies show that soy foods do not increase cancer risk, and may lower certain types of cancer.[30] Asian populations typically do eat more soy, however, and they typically have a lower incidence than Western populations.[31]

Prostate Cancer and Men's Health

Some speculation on soy's effect on men has circulated again due to the phytoestrogens in soy. However, in cell and animal studies, soy has been shown to decrease tumor growth and increase self-destruction of prostate cancer.[32,33] Furthermore, Asian countries historically have the highest rates of soy intake and lowest rates of prostate cancer, in stark contrast to Western countries. Chinese and Japanese men who immigrate West and forgo their soy staple diet fare much worse than their counterparts who still consume traditional foods after the move.[32]

Cancer Survivors

The American Institute for Cancer Research highlights soy as one of its "Foods that Fight Cancer." Many population studies indicate a significant correlation between dietary soy intake and lower instances of cancer.[33]

Other prospective studies have noted a decrease in cancer recurrence with higher soy intake.[31,34] The fiber in soy can also reduce the risk of colorectal cancers.[33]

The body of literature on soy doesn't seem conflicting when carefully examined. However, the bad press soy receives is often due to either a misinterpretation of research or references early studies that used isolated forms of soy or high-dose supplements. The research mentioned above tracked dietary soy and indicated that intakes two or three times greater than typical allotments are still safe and beneficial to one's health.[33] Ultimately, we recommend choosing more whole-food-based forms of soy, not isolated or supplemental forms. Whole-food forms of soy include edamame (baby soybeans), soybeans, soymilk, tofu, tofu noodles, soy nuts, soy yogurt, miso, and tempeh. Texturized soy protein (also known as texturized vegetable protein or TVP), soy protein isolate, and soy protein powder can be healthy, but pay attention to additional ingredients added. These altered forms of soy are often found in processed food products. Read the label and make sure it's a healthy and balanced product.

Hypothyroidism

Some research has suggested that soy can make hypothyroid medications less effective. However, this doesn't mean to completely avoid soy foods. Awareness and education with medication timing can help prevent and avoid potential negative effects. Ideally, you would maintain your normal intake of soy, and your doctor can adjust your medication dose to your diet. For patients who have subclinical hypothyroidism, it has been called into question whether soy can move them to diagnostic criteria.[35] It appears that iodine status also plays an important role; people with adequate iodine intake may not exhibit the symptoms that those with subclinical hypothyroidism and low iodine do.[36] If you're having problems with energy levels, temperature regulation, and/or weight gain, talk to your doctor about checking your thyroid levels using the proper testing to get an accurate and helpful diagnosis. Also keep in mind that sea salt does not contain iodine, so if you're cooking a lot of whole foods with minimal processing, consider using iodized table salt since it's fortified. Check your salt – popular brands may not be iodized.

FOOD FEATURE: TOFU'S STORY

You've heard tofu doesn't have any taste? Well, neither does flour before adding other ingredients and baking it! One of the benefits of tofu is its neutral flavor. It will take on the taste of what you cook or blend it with. Crumble it up in meat dishes, add it to smoothies, blend with ricotta, or make it center stage like in a tofu and veggie stir-fry.

TOFU FACTS:

- A vegan source of complete protein – yep, that means it's got all the same essential amino acids as beef!
- 25% DV for calcium in ½ cup[37]
- Lowers LDL cholesterol and blood pressure[38]
- Just ½ cup is a good source of iron, copper, and magnesium[33]
- Excellent source of selenium and manganese in ½ cup[33]

FIT TIP:

If you're an avid runner, add some tofu and a good source of vitamin D, like mushrooms, into your regular diet for a boost for bone health. Look for mushrooms that have been exposed to UV light – they'll be labeled as a good source of vitamin D. Cook them up together with soy sauce, olive oil, balsamic vinegar, and garlic for a great post-run recovery meal.

Nuts, seeds, and whole grains

Nuts and seeds are composed of carbohydrates, proteins, fats, fiber, and many vitamins and minerals like magnesium. They can be simple yet nutrient-packed additions to smoothies, dips, spreads, and breading, which can help boost heart healthy fats (alpha-linolenic acid, etc.) and protein. They are a calorie-dense protein option since they contain fat and carbohydrates too, so keep this in mind with your meal selections to properly meet your needs. They have also been highlighted as great options to prevent the risk of heart disease and diabetes. We'll be giving you more of a lowdown on nuts, seeds, and whole grains later on in the fat section.

Melissa Halas MA, RDN, CDE

Plant-based milks

While dairy products naturally contain protein, not all dairy substitutes contain the same nutrition profile. Today, plant-based milks are in abundance, giving you several options to choose from. Get in the habit of taking a glance at the nutrition facts label on the milk you choose, especially if you're looking for a calcium or vitamin D boost. We've compiled a list **(1.1 - Milk Comparisons for 1 Cup on page 22)** of some common brands and what you can expect from them. We also included cow's skim milk so you can see how it compares.

Protein Quality

Plant-based proteins contain different amounts of amino acids, which is why they vary in quality. Proteins differ in how available they are to us based on their digestibility, which depends on their food source. This means that the types and amounts of protein we consume, as well as the cooking methods, matter.

While you shouldn't feel like you have to memorize any definitions or values, the biggest takeaway from this section is to understand that there are different ways that protein quality is scored. It factors in how animal and plant proteins differ compared to one another and why it's important to have a variety of plant foods in your diet – especially if you're a vegan or vegetarian!

Don't feel like you have to understand it all at once – you can refer back to this section at any time.

Digestibility – Not All Proteins Digest the Same

Animal proteins

Animal proteins have higher digestibility than plant-based proteins, meaning their amino acids are absorbed better and at higher rates than those from plants.[20] In fact, the digestibility of animal proteins ranges from 90-100%, with meat and cheese at approximately 95%, and eggs at 97-100%.[20,39] In other words, 95% of the protein ingested from a specific serving of meat or cheese is digested by the body and available for absorption.

1.1 – Milk Comparisons for 1 Cup

Brand/milk type	Cals (kcal)	Pro (g)	Fat (g)	Sat fat (g)	Carb (g)	Sugar (g)	Fiber (g)	Calcium (mg)	Vit A (IU)	Vit D (IU)
Cow's milk, skim, with vitamins A & D	80	8	0	0	12	12	0	299	500	115
Ripple Foods pea milk, original, unsweetened	70	8	4.5	0	0	0	0	450	500	120
Silk soymilk, unsweetened	80	7	4	0.5	4	1	1	299	501	120
Pacific Naturals oat drink, original	130	4	2.5	0	24	19	2	350	500	100
Tempt Hemp milk, fortified, unsweetened	80	2	8	0.5	1	0	0	300	500	100
Silk almond milk, original, unsweetened	30	1	2.5	0	1	0	1	450	500	100
Silk cashew milk, unsweetened	25	1	2	0	1	0	0	450	500	100
Dream Blends, drink, rice & quinoa, enriched, unsweetened	60	1	2.5	0	9	1	0	300	500	100
Rice Dream, rice milk, original, enriched, unsweetened	70	0	2.5	0	11	1	0	250	500	100
Silk coconut milk, refrigerated, unsweetened	45	0	4.5	4	1	0	0	450	500	100

Source: ESHA Genesis R&D Software Version 11.5.1

Melissa Halas MA, RDN, CDE

Plant proteins

Plant-based proteins, such as legumes, have a lower digestibility range, between 70 and 90%.[20] This is because their protein content is encased in carbohydrate, making it more difficult for your body to get to the protein. However, this doesn't mean that all plant proteins aren't good quality. "Protein quality is determined by its essential amino acid composition and the digestibility and bioavailability of its amino acids."[40] Cooked split peas' digestibility is around 70%, and that of some soy-based products like tofu have a higher value of approximately 90%.[20,41]

NUTRITION TIP

Black beans have just as many antioxidants as acai, so maybe we should start calling black beans a "superfood"! They also have a minimal eco footprint. When purchasing plant-based foods, think local!

Biological Value

Another characteristic that contributes to a protein's quality is its biological value. Most animal proteins are high in biological value, while plant-based proteins are lower. Biological value refers to how much nitrogen in a particular protein the body is able to absorb and utilize for practical purposes, such as growth and repair.[20]

- The body is, for example, able to retain 94% of the nitrogen from eggs, hence its high biological value of 94.[39] Think of this measure of how efficient the body is at using the protein in that food.
- Biological value is calculated with an equation that accounts for the amount of nitrogen in the urine, the amount of nitrogen ingested from protein foods, and the amount absorbed.
- Values range on a scale of 0 to 100.
- While animal foods have higher biological values than those of plant-based foods, soybeans are a great plant-based protein option with a biological value of 72.8.[38]

While biological value is a useful measure for many proteins, there are other ways that protein quality is assessed. We won't be covering all of them, but let's take a closer look at a few of the key ones.

The Deeper Science on Protein Quality

 Eating a variety of plant-based foods or including eggs and/or dairy provides protein in a range of biological values. However, a small sector of competitive athletes are interested in detailed macronutrient planning. So for those who want to dig further, here's more science on protein quality. If you aren't part of this group, skip ahead to "Why eat plant-based proteins if most animal sources are higher quality?"

Protein Digestibility Corrected Amino Acid Score (PDCAAS)

Digestibility and biological value are two important factors to account for when trying to maximize protein intake and assess protein quality.

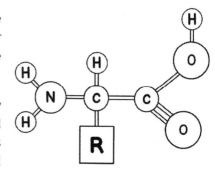

Another approach for protein quality is the Protein Digestibility Corrected Amino Acid Score (PDCAAS), which has been the standard used by the Food and Agricultural Organization (FAO), World Health Organization (WHO), and many other health professionals since 1991.[42] This score accounts for the amino acid content of the food item, as well as the percent true protein digestibility.[43]

- It is calculated by accounting for the limiting amino acid (the amino acid that's in suboptimal amounts) content and the digestibility of the protein.[44]
- Values from this method can range from 0 to 1.0. A score of 1.0 means that the food meets or exceeds the requirements for amino acids for humans – thus being a high-quality protein by the PDCAAS definition.

However, there have been key limitations with the PDCAAS from the beginning, one of which was the fact that the PDCAAS score is capped at a value of 1.00, even if high biological value proteins exceed this value in the calculation. It also calculates the values by total tract digestibility through fecal content, rather than absorption in the small intestine. "This is problematic since some of the nitrogen disappearance in the large intestine is due not to protein digestion and absorption, but rather to microbial degradation, resulting in ammonia production, absorption, and excretion as urine."[13] Ultimately, this means that high-quality proteins may be undervalued, and lower quality proteins could be shown as greater than they actually are. This is why newer research has been evaluating yet another method to test protein quality, the Digestible Indispensable Amino Acid Score (DIAAS).

Digestible Indispensable Amino Acid Score (DIAAS)

In 2011, the FAO proposed a new method called the Digestible Indispensable Amino Acid Score. This is meant to examine how amino acids are digested in a specific portion of the small intestine, the terminal ileum. It is proposed to be more accurate than the PDCAAS method because the process doesn't assume how the body is processing amino acids in the total gastrointestinal tract based on the total protein in that food.[42] This matters because amino acids are only metabolized in the small intestine, and some amino acids are not digested as well as others. Taking the amino acid content of a specific food without accounting for digestion in the terminal ileum doesn't give a true sense of how the body is processing and using the amino acids – also known as bioavailability.

Unlike the PDCAAS score, the DIAAS score is not capped at 1.00.[42] There are foods that are given a score of 1.00 on the PDCAAS scale that would have gotten a higher score without the cap. This makes the mechanism of evaluation for PDCAAS less accurate and as mentioned before, may underestimate the quality of some proteins. The DIAAS method removed this cap to aim for more accuracy. However, while the FAO would like the DIAAS to be the preferred method, more research is needed to fully implement it as the gold standard of protein quality.[42] Therefore, you don't see this value as commonly used, as many foods have not been studied, making their values unavailable.[44,45]

Evaluating PDCAAS and DIAAS scores

The values from DIAAS and PDCAAS can't be compared side by side, since they operate on different scales. When you're taking a look at the following chart, it is best to compare the foods within the DIAAS column without comparing to the PDCAAS column.

For competitive athletes, this can be helpful when looking at the quality of the proteins you are consuming throughout your day and/or week, or perhaps a plant-based supplement you were thinking about purchasing. We'll cover more about this in our supplement insights section.

In the section below, you will see several values for common plant-based foods/proteins and how they compare.

Here is an overview of different food sources and their digestibility, PDCAAS, and DIAAS values. Not all values have been established and the peer-reviewed values available can differ.

1.2 - Assessing Protein Quality			
Food	Digestibility (%)	PDCAAS	DIAAS (%)
Dairy Foods			
Cheese	95	1.00	
Eggs	97	1.00	113
Milk	91	1.00	114
Greek yogurt		1.00	
Skim milk protein powder	96	1.00	105
Milk protein concentrate	97	1.00	120
Whey protein concentrate	97	1.00	107
Whey protein isolate	96	0.97	100
Soy Foods			
Tofu	95.7	0.56	54
Edamame	90.5	0.95	
Tempeh	91.41 +/- 3.76		
Soy protein	95-98	1.00	
Soya flour	90	0.93	89
Soy protein concentrate	97	1.0	
Soy protein isolate	96 96-98 89.52	0.86 0.95-1.00	84
Legumes			
Black beans	78	0.75	
Chickpeas, canned	85	0.71 0.52	83
Pinto beans, canned	78	0.59	
Lentils	88-91	0.52	
Pea protein concentrate	94	0.71	62
Peanuts	94	0.52	

Melissa Halas MA, RDN, CDE

1.2 - Assessing Protein Quality (Continued)			
Food	Digestibility (%)	PDCAAS	DIAAS (%)
Other			
Oatmeal	86		
Wheat, whole	86	0.50	45
Rice	88	0.62	59
Corn	85		
Meat and fish	94		
Chicken breast		1.00	108

Sources: 44.45.49.48.46.50.48.52.53.54.55.56.40.47

Why eat plant-based proteins if most animal sources are higher quality?

Yes, animal proteins may score higher on the quality scales, but that doesn't mean they're healthier. Plant-based proteins are packed with other quality ingredients, such as vitamins and minerals, essential for optimal performance, and fiber and phytochemicals, important for disease prevention and overall health. More of these benefits are discussed later. Animal proteins don't have the same benefits due to their lack of both fiber and phytochemicals. Therefore, by substituting some of your animal protein with plant-based proteins you will reap short- and long-term health benefits, while still getting the amino acids you need for your workouts.

PROTEIN TIP

Leucine can help maximize your workouts because it triggers protein synthesis, which means it helps kick-start the mechanism to rebuild muscle and can contribute to muscular adaptations.

Branch Chain Amino Acids (BCAAs)

Leucine, isoleucine, and valine make up the branch chain amino acids (BCAAs). They are "special" because they don't need to go through the liver before being metabolized; they go straight into the bloodstream. While leucine gets all the attention for muscle building, all three of these essential amino acids work together for optimal muscle protein synthesis. Not getting adequate amounts of any of them can have a negative impact on muscle growth and maintenance. And it doesn't stop there. Research has shown that consuming a high-quality meal with all of the essential amino acids (all nine!) has a more pronounced muscle building effect than just the BCAAs alone.[57]

You have likely seen many pre-workout supplements or BCAAs in powder form. There is still limited research on the effectiveness of taking them before or during exercise. If you do consume a mixture of BCAAs, aim to consume it after your workout. Or, better yet, just eat adequate protein consistently.

If you are reaching your protein needs each day, BCAA supplementation likely won't provide a performance benefit.[58] The key thing to keep in mind is that you require all of the essential amino acids for muscle building, so it's best to consume protein sources with adequate leucine and complete (or close to complete) protein whenever possible.

The Lowdown on the Amino Acid Leucine

Leucine is one of the essential amino acids that has often been mentioned in the sports nutrition circle and investigated in research related to muscle protein synthesis. Leucine appears to act as a "trigger" or "switch" that turns on muscle protein synthesis in our muscles.[59] Additionally, it has a mediating role in increasing anabolism (growth) by increasing the transport of other amino acids into muscles. This increases the muscles' amino acid pool.[41] Muscles can then draw on the amino acids in the amino acid pool to assimilate, rebuild, and repair muscle tissue.

Leucine is highest in dairy protein, specifically whey protein, which is why you may hear that whey protein is optimal after a workout.[60] This is true, but plant-based protein sources can also be high in leucine if ingested in higher amounts. A dose of about 1-3 grams of leucine appears to be the optimal amount to trigger muscle protein synthesis.[57] Older adults may need closer to 3-4 grams per meal because muscles are not as responsive to protein/amino acids as a result of the aging process.[48,61]

You can mix and match the foods in Chart 1.3 to reach the highest amount of leucine. Check out the protein powder section later in the book for more about leucine in powders.

1.3 - Leucine Content In Foods	
Food	Leucine content (g)
1¼ cups tempeh	2.97
1½ cups white beans, canned	2.51
1½ cups red kidney beans, canned	1.84
1½ cups black beans, canned	1.84
¾ cup firm tofu	1.49
3 cups skim milk	2.34
1 cup plain, nonfat Greek yogurt	2.15
3 eggs, whole, cooked, poached	1.62
1 cup cottage cheese, nonfat	1.50

Source: USDA Food Composition Database[65]

Ten Quick & Easy Meals and Snacks to Maximize Muscle Growth

- Breaded tofu bites (*see the companion recipe book*) with 2 clementines
- Chopped tempeh with quinoa and dressing
- Stir-fry with edamame, vegetable mix, and brown rice
- Black bean, corn, and edamame salad
- Mango, kale, black bean and quinoa salad
- Small corn tortilla with 1 egg, kidney beans, salsa, cumin and paprika
- One cup low-fat cottage cheese with fruit + granola – pineapple tastes great!
- Smoothie with a fruit of choice, whey, pea or soy protein powder or Greek yogurt, and almond milk
- Greek Yogurt Bowl – nonfat plain Greek yogurt with cherries, almonds, and cocoa powder
- Tuna Wraps – tuna salad made with corn, tomato, and celery, mixed with quinoa, put into lettuce wraps

FIT TIP

If muscle and strength gain is a goal you are going for, then be sure to include a leucine-rich food most days in your post-workout snack or meal.

Keep in mind that in plant-based meals, you may need more than average protein per meal to meet the recommended leucine amounts. "Most plant-based sources have a leucine content of ~6-8%, whereas animal-based protein sources tend to have a leucine content in the range of ~8-9%, but >10% in the case of dairy proteins."[63,64] This is why you need to eat a larger serving of plant-based sources of leucine. But don't forget these plant-based sources also offer phytonutrients, fiber, vitamins, and minerals that animal sources don't have.

NUTRITION TIP

Not crazy about tofu? Meet yourself halfway – if you like smooth textures, opt for soft or silken tofu to add to soups and stews. For a denser substitution for dishes like burger patties or stir-fry, use firm or pressed tofu. If you're making bean or meat tacos, add in some crumbled tofu cooked with chili powder and salsa. You'll still have the taste and protein you want, with the addition of powerful phytochemicals.

Protein Myth-Busting: Complementary Plant-Based Proteins

Complete proteins are foods that contain an adequate amount of each of the nine essential amino acids needed by the body – remember the chart we showed you earlier? Most plant-based proteins are too low in one or two of the essential amino acids to be considered complete proteins, so they are *incomplete proteins*. However, there are a few exceptions to this, such as soy protein, quinoa, and chia seeds – they are *complete* proteins. Even though they may be complete, they may be low in one of the essential amino acids. For example, soy is lower in methionine than animal proteins. This is why it's essential to eat a variety of plant-based proteins throughout the day.

It used to be commonly thought that in order to get all of the essential amino acids in the amounts needed by the body, vegetarians and vegans needed to consume complementary plant-based proteins together at each meal in order to create complete proteins. We now know that it is **not** necessary to consume complete protein combinations at every meal. In fact, it's best to get your protein throughout the day instead of concentrating it in one or two meals. Proteins with different essential amino acid concentrations can be consumed throughout the day in order to adequately provide the body with all of the essential amino acids it needs. However, you can mix different plant-based proteins at meals if you want a higher quality protein mix. For example, legume protein is higher in lysine and lower in sulfur amino acids than wheat, which has the opposite profile. Combining these together is an example of how to reach a higher protein quality meal.[40] The varying amino acids consumed from balanced and diverse meals throughout the day will contribute to the amino acid pool, and the body will draw on this pool to synthesize proteins.

NUTRITION TIP

Avoid getting a majority of your daily protein intake in one or two meals. Instead, strive to add a source of plant-based protein during each meal and snack consumed.

FOOD TIP

Note that hummus, a popular plant-based protein, only has 1 gram of protein per 2 tablespoon serving. Don't let this stop you from eating it, because it can add a ton of flavor to grains and veggies! However, just make sure you're not counting it as your primary protein source at that meal.

A Closer Look at Sources of Plant-Based Protein[20]

As you have learned, plant-based protein foods are foods that aren't sourced from animals. While dairy products are animal-based, they can serve as important non-meat sources of protein for vegetarians – with an added bonus of being naturally high in calcium. They can also serve as a method to boost fruit and veggie intake, such as dips made with veggies and yogurt, or smoothies made with fruit and yogurt. Greek, Nordic, and Icelandic yogurts are typically higher in protein than traditional yogurt.

Using a tasty protein-rich sandwich spread, dip, or dressing can help you meet your protein goals. Try this Greek dressing/yogurt dip to go with cut up veggies or add in a little extra olive oil and whisk it all together to make a dressing to go with your protein-packed salad.

Ingredients:

- 1 cup nonfat Greek yogurt
- 2 teaspoons sweetener of choice (try sugar, honey, maple syrup, or agave)
- 2 teaspoons acid (such as lemon juice, white vinegar, or apple cider)
- 1 teaspoon flavored mustard (spicy mustard, Dijon or honey mustard)
- 1 teaspoon combo of your favorite herbs and spices (we love smoked paprika, cumin, and chili-lime seasoning)

Try eating savory yogurts as a snack. Mix 1 cup of yogurt with ½ teaspoon of each onion powder and garlic powder, and 2 teaspoons of lemon juice (preferably Meyer for their sweeter taste). Then add in a few tablespoons of your favorite fresh, chopped herbs. Sprinkle in salt and pepper and enjoy. It's delicious!

1.4 - General Averages of Protein and Fiber in Grains, Legumes, and Dairy			
Food	Serving size	Protein (g)	Fiber (g)
Greek yogurt	1 cup	26	0
Tofu, cubed	1 cup	27	2
Lentils, cooked	1 cup	18	16
Chickpeas/ garbanzo beans	1 cup	15	13
Seitan, cubed	¼ cup	15	1
Tempeh (soy based)	3 oz.	16	7
Bean pasta, cooked	1 cup	12	5
Beans, cooked (black, kidney, white, or pinto)	1 cup	15-17	11-15
Whole wheat bread	1 slice	4	2

Source: USDA Food Composition Database[62]

Nuts and seeds have a place any time of the day. Try tossing them in salads, eat them as nut and seed butter (pumpkin seed butter), add a spoonful of some ground flax seeds into a smoothie, or experiment with chia seeds. These are good for smoothies, pudding, jams, or as an egg substitute.

FOOD TIP

For quick and easy plant-based egg substitutes, give one of these a try:
- 1 tablespoon Chia seeds, soaked in 3 tablespoons water
- 1 tablespoon ground flax seeds, soaked in 3 tablespoons water

1.5 - Protein and Fiber from Nuts & Seeds for 100 Calorie Portions[65]

Nut or Seed	Serving size	Protein (g)	Fiber (g)
Hemp seeds	2 Tbsp.	6	1
Pumpkin seeds (pepitas)	2 Tbsp.	4	1
Peanuts	17 nuts	4	1
Almonds	14-15 nuts	4	2
Pistachios	25 nuts	4	2
Sunflower seeds	2 Tbsp.	4	2
Sacha inchi	2 Tbsp.	4	1
Flaxseeds (ground)	2 Tbsp.	3	3
Cashews	11 nuts	3	1
Chia seeds	1 Tbsp. + 1 tsp.	3	7
Brazil nuts	3 nuts	2	1
Hazelnuts (filberts)	11 nuts	2	2
Pine nuts	2 Tbsp.	2	1
Walnuts (whole)	4 nuts (8 halves)	2	1
Pecans (halves)	10 nuts	1	1
Macadamia nuts	5.5 nuts	1	1
Chestnuts	4 nuts	1	2

Source: USDA Food Composition Database[62]

1.6 - Protein and Fiber from Nuts & Seeds for 1 Tablespoon Portion[62]

Peanuts, tree nuts, & seed butters	Protein (g)	Fiber (g)
Peanut	3.5	1.0
Almond	3.5	1.5
Cashew	3.0	0.5
Sunflower	3.0	1.0
Sesame	2.5	1.0
Macadamia	2.0	1.0

Source: USDA Food Composition Database[62]

FOOD FEATURE: CHIA SEEDS

Cha-cha-cha chia! If you recognize that song, you've just dated yourself! Chia seeds once known for the Chia Pet, might start appearing as a thickener and emulsifier in foods. Great news for those whose guts are sensitive to guar gum!

CHIA SEED FACTS:
- A vegan source of complete protein[66]
- 20% protein by weight[66]
- Gram for gram, chia seeds have more calcium than milk! (631 milligrams calcium/100 grams of chia, 143 milligrams calcium/100 grams of milk)[62]
- It's likely you're not going to have 100 grams (3.5 ounces of chia) in one sitting, nor is that recommended. But 2 tablespoons of chia seeds do have 179 milligrams of calcium, making them a good source for a calcium boost to smoothies, breakfast cereal, or yogurt.[62]
- You can replace eggs in vegan baking by adding 1 tablespoon of chia seeds to 3 tablespoons of hot water.
- Provides an omega-3 boost through 5 grams of alpha-linolenic acid (ALA) with 2 tablespoons[62]
- Two tablespoons are an excellent source of soluble fiber – they can absorb more than ten times their weight in liquid!

FIT TIP:
Trained hard today? Add chia seeds to your post-workout snack! They can help lower inflammation with their alpha-linolenic compounds; plus, they're packed with fiber, which may help lower your risk of osteoarthritis – especially in the knees.

Proteins of the Future

Obtaining 1 pound of animal protein requires about 7.5 pounds of plant proteins, which are consumed by the animal as it grows. It's estimated the world population will reach 9.5 billion by 2050.[67] It will be unsustainable to meet the world's protein needs with our current diet. Meatless Monday is growing in popularity and more people are opting to increase the number of plant-based meals enjoyed per week. Innovative plant-based proteins are currently being studied throughout the world, and veggie burgers like the Impossible Burger and Beyond Burger are going mainstream at fast food restaurants. These plant-based options are enjoyed for their great taste and meat-like texture. Be on the lookout for even more options to come. Microalgae is a complete protein like spirulina that can contain up to 70% protein in dry weight. Duckweed, referred to as water lentils by some food scientists, is another potential source of low-cost plant-based protein for the future. Although it can be an invasive plant as it can double its size in less than 16 hours, when grown in a controlled environment it could serve as a sustainable high protein source for the growing population. It is also high in carotenoids, thiamin (vitamin B1) and pantothenic acid (vitamin B5).[68] Seaweed extracts are also being explored as a protein powder of the future.[67] One such seaweed, a strain of dulse, mimics the taste of bacon.[69] All of this effort is bound to show results for a more sustainable future.

The Protein Basics for Maximizing Muscle Gains & Maintaining Good Health

So, you know which foods contain protein, but how much should you actually be eating? This section covers protein needs specific to activity level so that you can see which category you fall into. While eating sufficient protein is important for muscle protein synthesis, there are many other important roles protein takes on for the active individual. Making sure you have enough protein can decrease your risk of injury and illness and improve your ability to train at the level you would like to be training. Now let's figure out how you can do that.

You do lose small amounts of protein in your urine and sweat, but keep in mind that less than 5% of the energy you use during exercise is from protein.

When researchers and sports dietitians evaluate nutrition needs for protein (and usually the other two macronutrients, carbohydrate and fat), they talk about protein needs in grams per kilogram (g/kg) of body weight. So, it's important to note that 1 kilogram (kg) is equal to 2.2 pounds (lb.) for your conversions.

How to Calculate Your Body Weight in Kilograms (kg):
Female Example: A 140-pound woman weighs 63.6 kilograms
140 lb. ÷ 2.2 lb./kg = 63.6 kg

If it's determined by a dietitian or health professional that this athlete needs 1 gram of protein per kilogram body weight per day, she would need 64 grams of protein per day.

Step 1: Assess Fitness Level

People have unique protein needs based on their level of fitness. The first step in deciding this fitness level is to figure out the metabolic equivalents that correspond with the intensity of exercise. Sometimes exercises overlap; for example, swimming, weight lifting, and practicing yoga on the same training day or a day of hybrid-like circuit training. To determine these needs, dietitians usually use a combination of factors. The guide below is just a snapshot.

Metabolic equivalent, or MET, is an index used to describe the intensity of an activity. For example, an activity with a MET value of 5, such as speed walking, would require 5 times the oxygen (and thus, energy) than that of a person at rest (i.e., sitting quietly, 1 MET).[70,71]

This is also how calorie expenditure is calculated. To put things into perspective, 1 MET = 1 kcal/ kg /hr. So, if the female from above was exercising at a moderate level (5 METS) for 1 hour, we would calculate her calorie expenditure as follows, finding the value for calories, x.

$$5 \text{ MET} = \underline{x}\text{ kcal} / 63.6 \text{ kg} / 1 \text{ hour}$$
$$5 \text{ MET} \times 63.6 \text{ kg} \times 1 \text{ hour} = \textbf{318 kcals per hour}$$

1.7 - Energy Expenditure Examples
Sedentary 1.0-1.5 METs
Defined as sitting, lying down, and expending very little energy
Moderate activity 3.0-6.0 METs (3.5 to 7 kcal/min)
<ul><li>Walking at a moderate or brisk pace of 3.0 to 4.5 mph on a level surface inside or outside, such as:<ul><li>Walking to class, work, or the store</li><li>Walking for pleasure</li><li>Walking the dog</li><li>Walking as a break from work</li><li>Walking downstairs or down a hill</li><li>Racewalking—less than 5 mph</li></ul></li><li>Using crutches</li></ul> <ul><li>Hiking</li><li>Roller skating or in-line skating at a leisurely pace</li><li>Light calisthenics or lighter weight lifting</li><li>Mowing the lawn (power mower)</li><li>Gardening (digging, raking, weeding)</li><li>Aerobic dancing</li><li>Golf (carrying clubs)</li></ul>

1.7 - Energy Expenditure Examples (Continued)
Vigorous activity Greater than 6.0 METs (more than 7 kcal/min)

- Mountain climbing, rock climbing, rappelling
- Roller skating or in-line skating at a brisk pace
- Bicycling more than 10 mph or bicycling on steep, uphill terrain
- Stationary bicycling—using vigorous effort
- Intense calisthenics or heavy weight lifting
- Exercise classes (spin, interval training)
- Moderate pick-up basketball
- Jumping rope (> 66 jumps/min)

Adapted from the Center for Disease Control and Clinical Cardiology[71,72]

You may do exercises of both intensities, so apply the category that best defines your average workout intensity. For more examples of exercises, see the chart referenced above.

Step 2: Select Protein Needs Based on Activity Level

Protein needs vary greatly based on lifestyle. If you're interested in getting an idea of your own intake, you can try spending a few days counting your daily protein intake then averaging it. This makes it easier to see if you're generally meeting your protein needs. Once you establish a basic understanding of your eating patterns, you don't need to continue to count protein grams, and instead, can re-evaluate every couple of months or when your training schedule changes.

Protein needs of sedentary people

The average sedentary person needs 0.8-1.0 grams of protein per kilogram of body weight per day. This should result in a minimum of 10% of an adult's daily energy intake from protein.[73]

Remember that this is in kilograms, NOT pounds.
To figure out how many kilograms a person weighs, again,
divide his or her weight in pounds by 2.2 (2.2 pounds = 1 kilogram).

Protein needs of athletes and exercise enthusiasts

Protein needs for more active individuals takes into account the higher demand on the body and the importance of preventing muscle breakdown, maintaining or promoting positive nitrogen balance, and supporting muscle protein synthesis.

1.8 - Protein Needs for Athletes and Exercise Enthusiasts		
Type of athlete or goal	Daily protein target (gram of protein/ kg body weight)	Additional information
Sedentary person	0.8-1.0	Older adults may be higher on this range.
Moderately - vigorously active	1.2-2.0[70]	Higher amounts may be required for athletes with high volume intense training. Includes team sport athletes.
Endurance	1.2-1.4[86]	
Strength	1.6-1.7[86]	
Resistance-trained athletes: Building/ maintaining muscle mass	1.4-2.0[57]	
Competitive bodybuilding	1.2-2.2[74] or up to 3 (Amounts >3.0 may have positive effects on body composition – more research needed)[74,75]	The first range appears to be sufficient if an athlete is at or above energy needs. No consensus, but some research shows higher amounts can be beneficial.
Resistance-trained athletes on a hypocaloric diet to maintain lean mass OR competitive bodybuilders during contest preparation	2.3-3.1 g of protein per kg fat-free body mass[57,74]	Greater than 3.0 g of protein/ kg of total body weight may have additional benefits for body composition.

Most moderately and vigorously active people fall into the 1.2-2.0 grams of protein per kilogram of body weight per day range. An exercise enthusiast working out at least 6-8 hours a week, including at least 2 days of muscle-strengthening activities that are moderate or high-intensity, could fall into a similar protein range. These activities can involve all major muscle groups, with protein needs ranging from 1.2-2.0 grams of protein per kilogram of body weight per day. However, keep in mind that there are many variations and types of weekly exercise routines, which is why there is a wide range of protein needs.[7,76]

Endurance and strength athletes need anywhere from 1.2-2.0 grams of protein per kilogram of body weight (BW) per day.[59,77-79] Endurance athletes are typically on the lower end of the spectrum at 1.2-1.4 grams of protein per kilogram of body weight per day, while athletes who are primarily doing resistance training will fall in the 1.6-1.7 grams of protein per kilogram of body weight per day range.[80] Exercise enthusiasts combining Pilates and/or weight training with cardio activities may also need 1.2-1.4 grams of protein per kilogram of body weight per day, depending on lean muscle mass gains desired. If your training regimen combines your primary sport (i.e., swimming) with strength training several hours per week, your protein needs will increase higher than endurance athletes. For athletes who are cutting calories or recovering from an injury, even higher protein amounts may be needed to protect their muscles from breakdown.[41,81]

For resistance-trained athletes who want to build or maintain lean muscle mass, most of them will fall in the range of 1.4-2.0 grams of protein per kilogram of body weight per day.[57] However, for someone who is doing resistance training and eating a hypocaloric diet (eating less than their needs) to cut weight, protein intake may increase further. The severity of the caloric deficit and type and intensity of training performed by the athlete will influence at what end of the range athletes choose to be.[79] They will likely fall somewhere between 2.3-3.1 grams of protein per kilogram of fat-free mass (FFM) scaled upwards with the severity of caloric restriction and leanness.[75,82]

Considering the range above, some bodybuilders may have higher protein needs greater than 3.0 grams of protein per kilogram of body weight.[57,82] Body builders should work with a dietitian with a sports nutrition background to determine if they're getting the right amount of protein while eating a diet that protects against heart diseases, cancer, or osteoarthritis, to minimize aging.

For highly competitive athletes, protein should be evenly distributed, every 3-4 hours a day, with high-quality protein when possible.[57] If you need a minimum of 1.6 grams of protein per kilogram of body weight per day, eating 0.4 grams of protein per kilogram of body weight per meal across a minimum of four meals will help reach your needs.[83] Likewise, if your needs are even higher, up to 2.2 grams of protein per kilogram of body weight per day you would need 0.55 grams of protein per kilogram of body weight per meal over four meals in the day.[83] These recommendations come from newer research examining the maximum amount of protein the body can absorb and utilize at one meal. More research needs to be done in this area, but these values can give you an idea of how you can spread out your protein maximize the value of your meals.

Research is evolving in protein muscle synthesis each year. You may see some conflicting research, for example, the recommendation of grams of protein per kilogram of body weight per day after exercising exceeding the typical recommendation of 20-25 grams of protein per meal. It is best to calculate your total needs and spread it throughout the day. For a higher body weight with higher protein demands, if you limit each meal to 20-25 grams of protein, you won't be able to meet your needs. Remember these are "guidelines" and plans need to be individualized.

Hydration concerns with higher protein intake

Fluid needs increase on higher protein diets as they can displace carbohydrate intake and raise the risk of dehydration. Carbohydrates, when stored in the muscle as glycogen, are also stored along with water, specifically 3 grams of water for every 1 gram of glycogen.[84] Therefore, if carbohydrate intake is inadvertently lower on a higher protein diet, less water is stored in the muscles and an individual should increase fluid intake to prevent dehydration. When on a high-protein diet, a person may not feel thirsty so monitoring adequate hydration is important.

Diets high in animal protein can also lead to constipation if not consumed with adequate water, carbohydrate, and fiber. This is yet another reason why plant proteins are so great – they naturally have fiber-rich carbohydrates, protein, and can contain some water.

EAT YOUR WATER

Adding vegetables to your meals and snacks boosts hydration while also meeting fiber needs to help promote regularity.

- cucumber: 96% water – perfect with white beans and homemade dressing
- celery: 95% water – yummy chopped in Greek yogurt dip
- radish: 94% water – crunchy sliced in salad bowls
- tomatoes: 94% water – sweet in tofu tacos
- cauliflower: 92% water – delicious to make into gnocchi

Example Calculations of Protein Needs

When doing the calculations below, always round your number up.

Female

Example: 140-pound female needing 1.2 g of protein/kg would need 77 grams a day

> Formula: 140-pounds ÷ 2.2 pounds/kg = 63.6 kg
> 63.6 kg × 1.2 g of protein = 77 g of protein per day

Example: 140-pound female needing 2.0 g of protein/kg would need 128 grams a day

> Formula: 140-pounds ÷ 2.2 pounds/kg = 63.6 kg
> 63.6 kg × 2.0 g of protein = 128 g of protein per day

So, depending on the needs of this athlete, if she falls within the 1.2 to 2.0 grams of protein per kilogram per day, she would have a range of 77-128 grams per day.

Male

Example: 180-pound male needing 1.2 g of protein/kg would need 99 grams per day

> Formula: 180-pounds ÷ 2.2 pounds/kg = 81.8 kg
> 81.8 kg× 1.2 g of protein = 99 g of protein per day

Example: 180-pound male needing 2.0 g of protein/kg would need 164 grams per day

> Formula: 180-pounds ÷ 2.2 pounds/kg = 81.8 kg
> 81.8 kg × 2.0 g of protein = 164 g of protein per day

So, depending on the needs of this athlete, if he falls within the 1.2-2.0 grams of protein per kilogram per day, he would have a range of 99-164 grams of protein per day. This is a pretty big range, so if you're fine-tuning your protein intake, expert guidance is recommended.

For reference, we've put together sample meal plans for an athlete or an exercise enthusiast that needs ~130 grams of protein per day so you can see how this would ideally look throughout the day.

1.9 - Sample Meal Plans - 100% Plant-based			
Meal	**Food**	**Plant protein in ingredients (g)**	**Total plant protein (g)**
Breakfast	½ scoop (~2 Tbsp.) pea protein powder	14	31
	½ cup rolled oats	3	
	1 oz. walnuts	4	
	½ cup frozen mango	0	
	½ cup soymilk	4	
	2 Tbsp. chia (pre-soak in soymilk)	6	
	Cinnamon	0	
Lunch	5 oz. tofu	14	34
	1 cup beans	14	
	3 cups stir-fry vegetables	6	
Snack	1 medium sized apple with a handful of almonds	6	10
	½ cup soy milk	4	
Dinner	3 oz. lentil pasta	21	53
	Served over 2 cups baby spinach with ½ cup marinara sauce	4	
	5 oz. cooked tempeh	28	
Total day protein			128

Meal	Food	Protein in ingredient (g)	Total protein (g)	Total plant protein (g)
1.9 - Sample Meal Plans (Continued) - Plant-based Protein Boost				
Breakfast	1 cup nonfat plain Greek yogurt	24	31	7
	½ cup rolled oats	3		
	1 oz. walnuts	4		
	½ cup frozen mango	0		
	Cinnamon	0		
Lunch	2 oz. chicken	14	34	20
	1 cup beans	14		
	3 cups stir-fry vegetables	6		
Snack	1 medium sized apple with a handful of almonds	6	12	6
	1 low-fat string cheese stick	6		
Dinner	3 oz. lentil pasta	21	53	25
	Served over 2 cups baby spinach with marinara sauce	4		
	4.5 oz. (cooked) salmon	28		
Total grams of protein			130	58

(See our companion book for more snack and meal ideas)

How Much Plant-Based Protein Should I Eat?

At first, your target should be to focus on boosting plant-based protein overall. If you don't already eat plant-based proteins, start by boosting one meal, then build your way up. If you already eat a mostly plant-based diet, then evaluate how many grams of protein you're getting in a day, and whether or not it's from a variety of sources (color, quality, and nutrients they provide).

People vary in their percentage of plant-based protein intake. It depends on personal lifestyle choices, health/family risk factors, and taste preferences.

Your diet should reflect your personal goals, should taste good and be enjoyable. Percentages can vary—some people eat 60% animal protein and 40% plant-based protein, while others could eat 50/50, 40/60, 70/30, and some eat all plant-based foods. Don't get hung up on percentages! Each person's needs and preferences are unique. There is no perfect or one-size-fits-all formula. Just remember, boosting plant-based protein has added health and environmental benefits, so no matter where you are, it helps.

Focus on total grams of protein and eating protein at each meal, then evaluate if you're getting the results you want with your training program and diet combined.

SHOPPING TIP

Buy bulk frozen salmon sealed in vacuum bags at a grocery store or club (Costco, Sam's Club, etc.). It's healthy and easy, plus a great source of omega-3s, which can decrease inflammation and help lower risk of heart disease.

Not getting results and unsure of what to change? Look for a Registered Dietitian (RD) or Registered Dietitian Nutritionist (RDN) –they're the same thing – who specializes in sports nutrition. These dietitians see athletes on a regular basis and have more experience with athletes than your typical dietitian. In addition, some RDs may be a CSSD (Certified Specialist in Sports Dietetics). They have a minimum of two years in the field of sports nutrition and are considered experts with this premier credential. However, some dietitians who already hold an additional credential, which requires annual continuing education units, may choose not to add the CSSD. Before hiring a dietitian, ask about their educational background, experience, and approach to sports nutrition. You can also find RDs with a background in exercise physiology or who are certified athletic trainers (ATC), as they will be more familiar with the demands of your exercise. They can help you put the puzzle pieces together to build the best diet for your unique training and performance needs.

PROTEIN ANALYSIS

Activity – Are you meeting your protein needs?

Your turn!

1. Calculate your protein needs using the information provided in the "Protein for Active Individuals" section.
   - You will need to know your weight and need to identify your activity level.

2. Keep a diet log for two weekdays and one weekend day. Add up your protein for each day* and assess if you are getting enough.
   - Check: Count how many times you included a plant-based protein source in your meals and snacks.

*Use a reliable source to quantify your protein intake, such as a product box or food label, online government website like the USDA Food Composition Database, Canada's eaTracker, or the Calorie Counter books by Simon and Schuster. Avoid publicly sourced online information for nutrition facts, or fitness trackers that pull from publicly sourced information. These can be highly inaccurate.

While we have a food-first mentality, we know that it can be tough to reach protein needs through food alone, especially with a hectic schedule and/ or with very high needs. For the 101 on protein powders, head to the section after Phytochemicals titled "Safety First With Supplements – How to Make Good Purchases."

Assessing Hydration Needs

We touched briefly on why hydration is important with increased protein intake, but as you can imagine, incorporating a fluid strategy throughout your day is just as important as making sure you're getting enough of the other essential nutrients. Our bodies are made up of between 45-75% water (crazy, right?!), and when we exercise, we need to make sure we're properly accounting for the fluid losses so we can rehydrate and stay in fluid balance.[80,85]

Water has many benefits including, but not limited to:

- regulating your body temperature
- removing wastes (i.e., urine, sweat, feces)
- lubricating and cushioning your joints

Proper hydration strategies are individualized and can be optimized by calculating or measuring your sweat rate and sweat composition. You can see a Registered Dietitian Nutritionist or an exercise physiologist to get more specific recommendations. However, in your day-to-day living, there are simple ways to make sure you are staying hydrated.

The WUT strategy is a simple way to account for three of the most important markers for hydration:[86]

- **W** stands for **Weight** – You can weigh yourself before and after a workout. For each pound you lose you need to rehydrate with about 16-24 ounces of water.[78]
- **U** stands for **Urine** – Monitor your urine color. Aiming for a pale-yellow, lemonade color is a simple way to stay on track.[87]
- **T** stands for **Thirst** – While you never want to rely solely on thirst as an indication that you need to drink fluids, it is a simple way (when combined with the other two factors) to know if you are doing a good job staying on top of your hydration strategy.

If two or more of these markers are present, dehydration is likely, and if all three are experienced, dehydration is *very* likely.[86]

A simple way to monitor these symptoms is to check your weight, urine, and thirst level at the start of each day. Your weight each morning shouldn't be changing by more than 1% from the previous morning (unless you are specifically aiming for certain weight goals), your urine should be a light color, and you shouldn't be thirsty. Keep a diary for a few days in order to identify any patterns.[86]

Hydrating During Exercise

While exercise lasting less than or equal to about 60-90 minutes shouldn't cause concern about electrolyte replacement in normal weather conditions, electrolyte replacement is something to be aware of for endurance activity or when in hot and humid environments or at high altitudes. For all levels of athletes, electrolyte replacement is important with the conditions above. For example, an exercise enthusiast hiking or mountain biking for over 90 minutes at a moderate pace in warmer weather may find that using electrolyte repletion improves their pace and decreases post-exercise fatigue.

Unfortunately, there isn't a one-size-fits-all approach for electrolyte and hydration strategies. Sweat rate and sweat content vary among individuals, which is why it's important to be aware of your body's response to different durations, types, and intensities of exercise. For example, if you're a salty sweater, you will need to take in more sodium than the average person. Not sure if you're a salty sweater? See if there is a white or colored salt ring (depending on the color of your clothes) of salty sweat around the inside of your hat or your t-shirt. This is key because rehydrating without proper amounts of sodium can lead to hyponatremia (when your blood and body fluids are diluted, and you don't have enough sodium to even out the losses.) This can have serious consequences, so it's important to have a strategy in place with your hydration, as you would with the rest of your nutrition. After all, water is one of the six classes of nutrients!

While you will often see sodium and potassium as two key ingredients in electrolyte replacement beverages, keep in mind that you lose a lot less potassium in your sweat than you do sodium. This means that you don't have to be quite as concerned about replacing potassium during exercise (unless you're doing an ultra-endurance event). Having a meal with adequate potassium after exercise should be enough to replace your losses.

Even though hydration strategies differ from person to person, and the total amount of fluid you have to consume during your exercise varies, there are general guidelines you can use as a starting point. For prolonged activity, here are the proposed amounts of nutrients to add to beverages to maximize your hydration strategy:[88]

1.10 - Hydration During Exercise		
Nutrient	**Recommended range**	**Conversion**
Carbohydrate	~5-10% carbohydrate	50-100 g carbohydrate/L
Sodium	~20-30 meq sodium/L (chloride as the anion)	460-690 mg sodium/L (conversion of sodium only)
Potassium	~2-5 meq potassium/L	78-195 mg potassium/L

Sports Beverage Composition and Recommendations

The following beverage options are an example of the common nutrient composition of typical sports drinks on the market today used for longer duration exercise. You will notice that Option 1 closely resembles the guidelines above.

Option 1: Sports drinks

A combination of carbohydrates and electrolytes are combined in water to make a sports drink that provides fuel and can help counter any electrolyte losses from sweat. The example ranges below are the amounts of each nutrient found in typical sports drinks on the market today.[89] The amounts relatively reflect research recommendations for drinks.

1.11 - Sports Drinks		
Nutrient	**Composition of common sports drinks provide**	**Conversion***
Carbohydrate	5-8% carbohydrate	50-80 g carbohydrate/L
Sodium	10-35 mmol sodium/L	230-805 mg sodium/L
Potassium	3-5 mmol potassium/L	117-195 mg potassium/L

*Notice these are based on 1 liter of fluid, so if you're buying a 500-milliliter sports drink, divide by half.

You can also evaluate powder supplements and add the amount of water required to get to this dilution.

Option 2a: Powdered hydration mix

Many of these mixes can be purchased in small packets. One packet is usually mixed with 16 ounces of water (500 milliliters). Each flavor differs slightly, but here is an example of a lemon-lime flavor packet and how it compares to the recommended ranges:[90]

1.12 - Powdered Hydration Mix		
Nutrient	**Recommended range for 500 mL fluid**	**One packet per 500 mL fluid**
Carbohydrate	5-10% carbohydrate (25-50 g carbohydrate/500 mL)	21 g carbohydrate/500 mL
Sodium	230-345 mg sodium/500 mL	380 mg sodium/500 mL
Potassium	39-98 mg potassium/500 mL	39 mg potassium/500 mL

As you see in the chart above, the amounts of carbohydrate, sodium, and potassium are close to the ranges from the recommendations but differ slightly. For example, the carbohydrate content is slightly lower than the recommended range (21 grams versus 25-50 grams), the sodium content is above the range (380 milligrams versus 230-345 milligrams), and the potassium is on the low end of the range (39 milligrams for the 39-98 milligrams range). You may not find products that match recommendations in exact amounts, but the above product is an example of one that would be close enough.

Option 2b: Powdered electrolyte mix

There are many brands on the market today that use non-caloric sweeteners in combination with electrolytes. This can be beneficial when electrolytes need to be replaced, but carbohydrate is not needed for the duration of the activity. However, keep in mind that for longer duration exercise that requires carbohydrate intake, this type of electrolyte drink would need to be paired with a carbohydrate source (i.e., gel, bar, chews, etc.). Many gel and carbohydrate products do provide electrolytes as well, so make sure you aren't going overboard on the total amounts.

1.13 - Powdered Electrolyte Mix		
Nutrient	**Recommended range for 500 mL fluid**	**One tablet mixed with 500 mL fluid**
Carbohydrate	5-10% carbohydrate (25-50 g carbohydrate/500 mL)	1 g carbohydrate/500 mL
Sodium	230-345 mg sodium/500 mL	300 mg sodium/500 mL
Potassium	39 - 98 mg potassium/500 mL	150 mg potassium/500 mL

Option 3: High-level electrolyte replacement supplement

This is another common option found on the market but is more targeted towards specific athletes. These could include athletes who participate in weight sports and require rapid rehydration after weighing in, ultra-endurance athletes who need an electrolyte replacement supplement, or athletes who need a post-exercise strategy when medium-to-large amounts of fluid and sodium have been lost.[89] Here are common amounts of the main nutrients seen in this type of beverage:[89]

1.14 - High-Level Electrolyte Replacement Supplement		
Nutrient	**Composition of common sports drinks**	**Conversion**
Carbohydrate	2-4% carbohydrate	20-40 g carbohydrate/L
Sodium	50-60 mmol sodium/L	1150-1380 mg sodium /L
Potassium	10-20 mmol potassium/L	391-781 mg potassium /L

Note that the carbohydrate amount in these beverages are typically lower than the usual sports drinks as these types of athletes will be getting carbohydrate from other foods. The sodium and potassium are also much higher than many common sports beverages. This is why it's important to identify your need based on your sport (intensity and duration), as well as your sweat rate, and then seek out the correct electrolyte supplement to meet your needs.

The most important thing, no matter the duration of exercise, is to be aware of the amounts of fluid you're losing from sweat, and how you're replacing them. If you're a heavy or salty sweater, you want to make sure you are replenishing with fluids and electrolytes to perform at your best. Making sure that you don't lose more than 2% of your body weight in a session is key, as this can be detrimental to your performance or health. It can lead to overheating and increase the risk of heat stroke.[78]

Rehydrating After Exercise

Consume 16-24 ounces of fluid per pound lost.[84,87] Remember, the goal here is to always replace the fluid that you lost during exercise. If you need a better sense of how much you lose, weigh yourself before and after, keeping track of the fluids you consume during that event, and if you urinated between the time you weighed in and weighed out.

Did you know that 99% of our sweat is water? We have two main electrolytes we lose in our sweat – sodium, and chloride. Other nutrients that we lose in minimal amounts include potassium, magnesium, calcium, iron, copper, zinc, nitrogen, amino acids and water-soluble vitamins.

The other electrolytes in our body fluids in addition to these are bicarbonate and sulfate.

These are all necessary for nerve impulses, to prevent cramps, and to make sure our muscles and heart can keep up with the demands of exercise.

HYDRATION TIP

Coconut water has been trending for a while and usually provides a good source of potassium. A typical 8-ounce serving has around 500 milligrams of potassium and around 10-15 grams of carbohydrate. If you're using coconut water to replete electrolytes and carbohydrates, pair it with a salty snack.

Part 2:
CARBOHYDRATES – YOUR BRAIN AND BODY NEED THEM

CARBOHYDRATES HAVE GOTTEN A BAD rap in recent years partly due to their exclusion in trendy fad diets. However, because they are the body's main source of energy and the primary energy source for your brain, carbohydrates are important to everyone – especially to athletes! Plant-based proteins are perfect to include for athletic performance because they contain both carbohydrates for energy and protein for muscle repair. In addition to animal-derived dairy products, plant-based carbohydrate sources include all fruits, vegetables, grains, and legumes. Carbohydrates also provide micronutrients that are crucial for metabolism, energy production, and red blood cell formation – all of which are essential for optimal athletic performance. Micronutrients are vitamins and minerals we need in trace amounts to be healthy; for example, vitamin E, iron, zinc, and iodine. On the most basic, elemental level, carbohydrates are composed of carbon, hydrogen, and oxygen.

The Best Choice of Carbohydrates Simplified

As you can guess, the best choice carbohydrates are fruits, vegetables, whole grains, legumes (beans and lentils), low-fat/nonfat milk, and unsweetened yogurt. These are whole foods that aren't refined, and they don't have added sugars. These all have accompanying nutrients that are beneficial for your body. There are three different types of carbohydrates: simple, complex and refined.

Simple Carbohydrates

Simple carbohydrates are short structures that are easy for the body to break down, including those in fruits, dairy products, and table sugars. These are called monosaccharides – which include glucose, fructose, and galactose – and disaccharides – sucrose (table sugar), lactose, and maltose. The simple carbohydrates can also come in the form of added sugar found in baked goods, treats, and other processed foods – which provide no additional health benefits besides energy in the form of calories and, of course, taste. Added sugars should be consumed in moderation, taking up no more than 5-10% of total calories in adults (for a 2,000-calorie diet, this equals 100-200 calories or 25-50 grams of added sugar). The World Health Organization (WHO) advises that consuming below 5% would provide additional health benefits.[91]

2.1 - Table Sugar Can Add Up Fast!	
1 teaspoon = 4 grams of sugar	
5.3 ounces flavored Greek yogurt has around 12 grams of sugar, equal to 3 teaspoons of sugar	
2 tablespoons of ketchup has 4 grams of sugar, equal to 1 teaspoon of sugar	
4 tablespoons of balsamic vinaigrette has 10 grams of sugar, equal to 2½ teaspoons of sugar	
15 whole grain little crackers (small, about half the size of saltines) has 4 grams of sugar, equal to 1 teaspoon of sugar	
Total sugar: 30 grams or 7½ teaspoons of sugar	

Don't be fooled – added sugar can add up quickly. In healthier, whole-food sources, simple sugars are accompanied by important vitamins, such as vitamin C in citrus fruits and minerals like calcium in milk or yogurt. These nutrients help an athlete's body function at its maximum potential.

Complex Carbohydrates

Complex carbohydrates are longer structures that take more time for the body to break down and absorb, preventing drastic rises and falls in blood sugar levels. They are considered polysaccharides because they have three or more carbohydrates in their chain. They are also great sources of fiber, which contributes to increased satiety, the feeling of being fuller, for a longer period of time. Complex carbohydrates include whole grains, starchy vegetables such as potatoes, sweet potatoes, and corn, as well as beans, lentils, and other legumes.

Refined Carbohydrates

Refined carbohydrates are those that have gone through a particular type of processing to remove the whole grain. Important nutrients and phytochemicals (lignan)/antioxidants (vitamin E, selenium) are located in the bran and germ. White bread, white rice, or white pasta undergo this kind of processing, stripping the food product of its natural nutritive portions, including fiber and many of the B vitamins. When you choose to eat white bread/white rice over a whole grain, you are only eating the endosperm, which means you are stripping yourself of the benefits (since the grain has been stripped of its benefits). It's ironic, because many food products will add these nutrients and more back in by fortifying the food product. Instead of keeping the original whole grain, all that remains is the basic starch that provides limited benefits to the body. While still longer in structure, the basic starch component breaks down rapidly. Unlike whole grains and other complex carbohydrates, these foods tend to cause blood sugar to spike and fall rapidly since it no longer contains the fiber. New research is showing that we are missing out on the benefits of not just whole grains, but resistance starch as well. Growing evidence is showing the detriment of ultra-processed foods and their association with chronic disease and mortality.[92]

Carbohydrates Have Three Important Roles in the Body

Carbohydrates Are the Body's Main Source of Energy

The body uses carbohydrates in the form of glucose to fuel its every movement and function. Ultimately, all types of carbohydrates are broken down by the body into glucose. The brain operates solely on this glucose unless under severe circumstances, such as a state of malnutrition or starvation. In these situations, the brain can rely on ketone bodies; however, it's not preferred as it is extremely inefficient over long periods of time. We can store glucose in the form of glycogen in our muscles and liver (more on this later).

Carbohydrates Are Muscle Sparing

This means that carbohydrates are used for energy in order to avoid breaking down muscle protein to meet the body's energy needs. Protein is needed to provide muscles with the substrates for muscle synthesis and repair (in addition to other bodily functions). Eating enough carbohydrate is just as important as getting enough protein for those trying to build muscle or improve performance.

Carbohydrates Are a Vital Part of Fat Metabolism

Without carbohydrates, fat cannot be metabolized and used by the body for a variety of essential functions. Remember this with the quote: "Fat burns in the flame of carbohydrates."

Choosing the Right Amount of Carbohydrates

While it is important for athletes to choose the right foods based on their sport, all athletes must ensure they are eating enough food to fuel their energy expenditure. Since carbohydrates protect the muscles against breakdown, athletes should be sure to consume enough throughout the day. In general, daily carbohydrate intake should be anywhere from 45-65% of daily calorie intake.[73] More sport-specific guidelines will be provided for specific body weight calculations later. Eating a snack or meal with carbohydrates is ideal after longer exercise in order to replace depleted muscle glycogen.

A Closer Look at Types of Carbohydrates

Whole Grains

Together with fruits and vegetables, whole grain sources of carbohydrates are the best choices for athletes in their overall eating pattern. A whole grain is a kernel that has ALL three of its original parts: the bran (most of fiber is found here), germ (most vitamins and minerals found here), and endosperm. Some grains have an inedible hull. Whole grains help athletes sustain their energy over longer periods of time while providing them with additional dietary protein.

Examples of whole grains include brown rice, quinoa, 100% whole grain bread, buckwheat, millet, amaranth, oats, rye, and barley, just to name a few. We'll dive further into these later with a breakdown of their nutrition profiles.

Key nutrients from whole grains – a brief overview of function

Whole grains also offer a host of vitamins and minerals which are important for your body, as they aid in the burning of fats, carbohydrates, and proteins.[19]

In addition to the basic functions listed below, there are additional benefits. For example, magnesium, a mineral that is often inadequate in the American diet, is important for asthma management, prevention of insulin resistance and hypertension, and heart health.[93] When you eat whole grains, these are the nutrients you will be eating and the roles they play.

2.2 - Key Nutrients from Whole Grains – A Brief Overview of Function	
Nutrient	**Function**
Iron	Delivers oxygen to cells and provides energy
Magnesium	Maintains normal muscle and nerve function, a healthy immune system, and participates in hundreds of enzyme reactions
Phosphorus	Builds strong bones and teeth and is essential for growth and repair of cells and tissues
Zinc	Plays a role in immune system defense
Copper	Forms hemoglobin, a protein in the blood that transports oxygen to the body's tissues and is vital in energy production
Manganese	Develops bone and tissue, helps in blood clotting, and activates important enzymes
Selenium	Functions as an antioxidant and plays a role in thyroid and immune function
B vitamins	Play essential roles in metabolism: Each B vitamin has its own function including healthy skin and muscle maintenance, nervous and immune system function, and formation of red blood cells

Source: National Institutes of Health, Office of Dietary Supplements[94]

NUTRITION INFO

Did you know the Food and Drug Administration (FDA) has tight regulations about the wording that can be used when referring to the amount of a certain nutrient in food? We've pulled together a cheat-sheet for you to reference if you're ever curious! **(2.3 - FDA Food Claims and Definitions on page 58)**

2.3 - FDA Food Claims and Definitions	
Claim	**FDA definition**
"excellent source of" "rich in" "high in"	Product contains 20% or more of the Recommended Dietary Allowance (RDA) for the specified nutrient in a standard serving size of the food
"contains" "provides" "good source of"	Product contains 10-19% of the RDA for the specified nutrient in a standard serving size of the food

RDA: Average daily level of intake sufficient to meet the nutrient requirements of nearly all (97%-98%) healthy people.
Source: The Food and Drug Administration (FDA)[95]

Highlighted whole grains

There are so many tasty benefits to whole grains that you can experiment with (gluten-free grains included). Explore these details on amaranth, barley, buckwheat/kasha, bulgur, corn, Kamut, millet, oats, quinoa, rice, rye, spelt, teff, wheat berries, whole wheat, and last but not least, wild rice.

Amaranth

Amaranth kernels are tiny – as small as poppy seeds. They have a crunchy texture and an earthy, herbal taste. The most available form of amaranth is the beige seed.[95]

In South America, amaranth is often sold on the streets and popped like corn. You can try the same by heating it in a skillet until the kernels pop into little white puffs (it takes practice to get it right!). Amaranth does not contain gluten, so it must be combined with flour to make leavened breads. It is used in breads, cereals, crackers, muffins, and pancakes. Try it as a hot cereal or in cornbread. It doesn't soak up all the liquid and expand significantly like rice, so if the directions say cook time is 20 minutes, don't think by cooking it longer it will absorb more liquid. You can cook and blend it to add to soup as a thickener or substitute some amaranth flour in cornbread.

Health benefits:
- A protein powerhouse! Amaranth is a plant-based, complete protein and contains lysine and methionine, amino acids that are missing in many grains.
- Amaranth is high in fiber and rich in calcium, iron, phosphorus, B vitamins, and vitamin E.

Barley

Barley has a particularly tough hull that you can't eat. You will most often see hulled barley, which retains more of the whole grain nutrients (minus a bit of the bran), but just takes a while to cook. Because barley's fiber is spread throughout the grain, even hulled, it's significantly higher in fiber than other whole grains. Pearled barley (paler and smaller in comparison to hulled barley) has lost all the germ and most of the bran which is not as nutritious as hulled barley.[96] For those that are intolerant to gluten, barley is one grain you will have to avoid since it contains a gluten protein called hordein. Barley is a hearty grain with a wide flavor spectrum that mixes well with all sorts of foods. It's excellent with soups and makes a great side dish.

Health benefits:
- The soluble fiber (beta-glucan) in barley is heart healthy because it helps lower cholesterol.[96]

FOOD FEATURE: BUCKWHEAT

Buckwheat soba noodles are a tasty addition to Asian dishes. They can help lower inflammation and cholesterol levels. It's a great starter whole grain noodle for those having a hard time making the transition from white rice noodles. Give it a try!

BUCKWHEAT FACTS:
- It's gluten free, despite "wheat" in its name.[97]
- It contains soluble fiber, insoluble fiber, and resistant starch.[97]
- One cup cooked groats (what the individual grain is called) is a good source of zinc.[62]
- It contains anti-inflammatory flavonoids.[97]
- It contains prebiotics.[97] Prebiotics are non-digestible carbohydrates that are fermented by probiotic bacteria in the lower gastrointestinal tract. This fermentation produces short-chain fatty acids which have many health benefits, including lowering the risk of certain types of cancer, improving gut health and enhancing calcium absorption.[98]

FIT TIP:
Give your gut a workout! With all three types of fiber and prebiotics, buckwheat can help you achieve optimal digestive health.

More On Buckwheat/Kasha

Buckwheat is triangular in shape and has a distinctive nutty flavor. The whole buckwheat kernel is known as a groat. Buckwheat flour is used to make soba noodles, which are widely popular throughout Japan and available at most U.S. grocery stores. Aside from being used as pasta, you can use buckwheat flour for pancakes too. Buckwheat has a greenish-ivory color, which is the untoasted form. It is also found in a reddish-brown color, which is known as kasha (toasted form). It's a great complement to mushrooms, salmon, and dill. Even though this has wheat in its name, it is not related to wheat, and it is gluten-free. Add buckwheat to your diet for its antioxidant and cholesterol-lowering properties.[99]

Health benefits:

- Buckwheat contains high levels of rutin (a flavonoid), which can reduce blood pressure, increase antioxidant ability, and has anti-cancer properties.[97]
- It's full of fiber! Buckwheat/Kasha provides soluble fiber, insoluble fiber, and resistant starch to make your gut happier![97]

Bulgur (wheat family)

Bulgur is wheat kernels (berries) that are boiled, dried, and then cracked. Since bulgur is already precooked and dried, it cooks very quickly – it takes only about 10 minutes! This grain is the perfect grain for those that want something that is quick and nutritious. Bulgur is great for making pilafs and salads. The best-known salad that uses this grain is tabbouleh – which is a dish loaded with fresh herbs – antioxidant powerhouses. There are different grinds, all of which cook quickly. The fine grind is used mostly for salads and is normally packaged in tabbouleh mixes. Coarse bulgur is normally used for pilaf or as a meat substitute in chili.

Corn

No matter which color it comes in – white, yellow, red, or blue – or which form – grits, polenta, corn tortillas, or popcorn – you are eating a whole grain that's naturally gluten-free. This grain is the only grain that is also eaten as a vegetable. There are so many ways to make corn dishes. See the companion recipe book for more ideas.

KAMUT® (wheat family)

Kamut® is a golden, slender grain that is twice the size and length of most wheat. It has a delicious, buttery taste and nutty flavor. Although it's been around for over a thousand years, it's relatively new in the American diet.

Kamut's trademark guarantees that it is grown on an organic farm, contains 12-18% protein and is the pure, ancient Khorasan variety of wheat. Among other specifications that may have higher polyphenol content, Kamut has a type of phytonutrient that can lower certain types of cancer risks and heart disease.[100-102]

Millet

Millet is small, round, and yellow in color, and is another gluten-free grain. It has a mild flavor and can become bitter if cooked incorrectly. To avoid the bitterness of cooked millet, toast it in ½ tablespoon of oil before boiling it. Toast at a lower heat when lightly browning millet, as it can begin to pop.

Oats

Next time you're food shopping don't pass up the oats! Many people like oats because of their naturally sweet flavor, which is why they are used in breakfast cereal, breads, cookies, and other baked goods. Oats are delicious and light when blended into flour and used in pancakes, waffles, or smoothies. No matter what type of oat you are buying (regular, quick, instant, or steel-cut oats), even though they go through minimal processing, they hardly ever lose their germ or bran. This is why all of the varieties can be considered whole grains. Beware of buying flavored instant oatmeal, because of the high amount of sugar and salt added. Check the ingredient list before your purchase instant oatmeal.

If you follow a gluten-free diet, pay attention! Some oats can become contaminated in manufacturing facilities that also process wheat, rye, or barley. An easy way to avoid this is to purchase gluten-free oats.[103]

Health benefits:
- Oats contain both soluble fiber, which helps lower your cholesterol, and insoluble fiber, which promotes digestive regularity.
- They have beta-glucan, a plant substance that helps lower cholesterol.
- Oats have high levels of antioxidants that will help protect your heart from the damaging effects of oxidizing LDL cholesterol.

FIT TIP

Bake your oatmeal in muffin tins for an easy breakfast that you can pack in your gym bag for a post-workout treat! See our tasty muffin cup recipes in the companion recipe book.

Quinoa

Quinoa is a very tiny bead-shaped grain that can come in many different colors such as ivory, red, and black, to name a few. Quinoa has a sweet, subtle, herbal taste. It is great as a base for salads, tasty in bean burgers, and good as an additional complete plant-based protein source. It can also be added into soups, baked goods, and of course, just eaten as a side dish. This is one of the few grains that really should be rinsed before cooking, as it contains a bitter taste because of the saponins on its surface if not rinsed. It is yet another gluten-free grain. If you don't have a colander with a tight enough mesh surface, use a flour sifter to keep the seeds from going through.

Rice

Brown rice is naturally gluten-free and is left whole with the bran attached. To make white rice, they go through a process called pearling, which involves removing the bran and germ from the brown rice. This causes the rice to lose more than half of the vitamins/minerals and all of the fiber. Brown rice has a nutty flavor and a chewier texture. It also takes longer to cook than white rice, but it's well worth it for all its benefits. If you are a fan of basmati or jasmine rice like I am (because of the fragrant aromatics and its long and slender shape), don't worry! You can also find brown basmati and brown jasmine rice. Check out red, purple and black rice too!

Health benefit:

Rice is easily digested and great for those who are gluten intolerant.

NUTRITION TIP

Rice & Arsenic

Arsenic is an element present in the environment from both natural and human sources. Health risks associated with long-term, high levels of arsenic exposure include higher rates of skin, bladder, and lung cancers, as well as heart disease.[104] Since arsenic resides in water, air, and soil, we might find arsenic in many foods that absorb it during crop growth, including grains, fruits, vegetables, and seafood.[105] Rice has higher levels of inorganic arsenic than other foods because it takes up arsenic from soil and water more readily than other grains.[104]

The FDA recommends that consumers can certainly eat rice as part of a well-balanced diet and should include different varieties with other grain foods to minimize potential adverse effects.[104] Consumer Reports recommends 4.5 servings per week of basmati rice from India, Pakistan, or California, or sushi rice; but limit yourself to 2 servings per week for other types of rice.

A serving size of rice is approximately 45 grams, ¼ cup uncooked or ¾ cup cooked.[106] To better plan your intake of rice, refer to the table and the point system created by Consumer Reports by visiting their site.[107]

Rye

You're likely familiar with rye bread, but have you ever thought of eating whole rye berries (kernels)? They are long, slender, and tan in color. If you do not like the strong flavor of rye, there is another form called triticale, which is a cross between rye and wheat. Rye is avoided in a gluten-free diet because it contains a gluten protein called secalin. This means that triticale should also be avoided on a gluten-free diet since it contains gluten too.

Health benefit:
Rye contains a fiber called arabinoxylan which is also a powerful antioxidant and can have a beneficial effect on the gut microbiota. This is only one of its many phytochemicals that have powerful benefits.[108,109]

Spelt (wheat family)
Spelt is a chewy grain that is similar to wheat berries. However, it is slightly larger and is a reddish color, with a milder flavor. Spelt can be used in place of wheat berries in most recipes. Spelt pasta offers a hearty taste and is delicious served with herbs and olive oil.

Teff
Teff grains, which are native to Ethiopia are extremely small – about 100 seeds are the size of one wheat kernel! Because teff is so small, it cannot be processed to remove the germ or bran. Therefore, all teff is considered a whole grain. Teff has a very pleasant, sweet flavor. It is normally found in a reddish-brown color. It can be used to make "teff polenta," a sweet breakfast porridge, or a savory side dish. It also can be ground into flour to be used in baked goods and is naturally gluten-free. You may see teff emerge as a gluten-free beer in the future.

Health benefit:
Teff is high in iron, calcium, and fiber – great for vegetarian or vegan athletes, or for those who have increased iron needs.[110,111]

WHAT'S A WHOLE GRAIN?

Per the Whole Grains Council, whole grains contain all the naturally-occurring nutrients of the entire grain seed in their original proportions. 100% whole grain means the bran, germ, and endosperm are present – the three components of a whole grain. Look for the 100% whole grain stamp on products.[112]

Wheat Berries
Wheat berries are whole wheat kernels with just the hull removed. They have the great flavor associated with wheat and can be used in any recipe, just like rice.

Whole Wheat

Whole wheat can be enjoyed in many different forms: whole wheat bread, pasta, pita, and tortillas, for example. When you buy any of these items, make sure to check the ingredient list to see that the first ingredient states WHOLE wheat, to enjoy the benefit of its nuttier flavor and nutritious benefits. Did you know there is also white whole wheat? It has a milder taste and the same basic nutrition profile, minus the phenolic compounds that provide its color.[113]

Wild Rice

Wild rice is not technically rice at all, but the seed of an aquatic plant. Wild rice is a long, slender grain with a dark black color. It has a strong flavor, which is why it is most often consumed in a blend with other kinds of rice. Make your own blend of brown rice and wild rice – it will look and taste wonderful.

2.4 - Whole Grains: Protein and Carbohydrate Content for ½-cup Serving of Cooked Grain[114]				
Grain	Protein (g)	Carbohydrate (g)	Fiber (g)	Fat (g)
Farro	6	30	3	0
Kamut	6	28	4	1
Spelt	6	26	4	1
Wheat, red	6	32	6	1
Cornmeal*	2	24	1	1
Steel-cut oats**	5	27	4	3
Rolled oats**	5	27	4	3
Amaranth*	4	19	2	2
Millet*	4	24	1	1
Quinoa*	4	21	3	2
Sorghum*	4	28	3	1
Teff*	4	20	3	1
Wild rice*	4	21	2	0
Buckwheat*	3	20	3	1
Bulgur	3	19	5	0
Couscous, made from durum wheat	3	18	1	0

2.4 - Whole Grains: Protein and Carbohydrate Content for ½-cup Serving of Cooked Grain[114] (Continued)				
Grain	Protein (g)	Carbohydrate (g)	Fiber (g)	Fat (g)
Forbidden rice*	3	34	2	1
Rice, brown*	3	26	2	1
Barley	2	28	4	0

Sources: USDA Food Composition Database[62], Whole Grain Council[114,115]

*Gluten-free grains

**Must purchase gluten-free oats

Simple cooking tips for whole grains

Add the recommended amount of water or broth and ½ -1 teaspoon salt (optional) to a 2-quart saucepan.[116] Add 1 cup of desired grain and bring to a boil.[116] Cover, reduce heat to low, and simmer for the recommended amount of time or until all of the water has been absorbed and grain is tender.[117] Turn off heat and let stand, covered, for 5-10 minutes. Fluff and serve.[116-118] Refer to the table below for specific instructions for different grains.

2.5 - Simple Cooking Tips for Whole Grains			
Grain (1 cup dry)	Water or broth in cups	Cooking time/ special instructions	Yield in cups
Amaranth	2½	Bring to a boil, cover, and simmer for 20 minutes.	2½
Barley, pearled	3	Bring to a boil, cover, and simmer for 45-60 minutes.	3½
Barley, hulled	3	Bring to a boil, cover, and simmer for 90 minutes.	3½
Brown rice	2½	Bring to a boil, cover, and simmer for 45 minutes. Let stand covered for 5 minutes.	3
Buckwheat, untoasted	2	Buckwheat is porous and will absorb water more quickly than other grains. For best results, bring water to a boil before adding buckwheat. Simmer for 20-30 minutes.	2½

2.5 - Simple Cooking Tips for Whole Grains (Continued)			
Grain (1 cup dry)	Water or broth in cups	Cooking time/ special instructions	Yield in cups
Buckwheat/ kasha, toasted	2	Bring to a boil, cover, and simmer for 15-20 minutes.	3
Bulgur, fine	1	Bring to a boil, cover, and simmer for 2 minutes. Let stand 5 minutes before draining excess water.	3
Bulgur, medium	1	Bring to a boil, cover, and simmer for 8 minutes. Let stand 5 minutes before draining excess water.	3
Bulgur, course	2	Bring to a boil, cover, and simmer for 20 minutes.	3
Corn grits	4½	Bring to a boil, cover, and simmer for 35-45 minutes.	4
Cornmeal	4	Add to boiling water, simmer on low for 20 minutes.	4
Whole grain Kamut®	3	If possible, soak overnight. Drain, add fresh water, simmer for 30-40 minutes. Un-soaked cook time is 40-60 minutes.	2
Millet	2¼	Bring to a boil, cover, and simmer for 20-30 minutes.	4
Oats, steel cut	4	Bring to a boil, cover, and simmer for 30 minutes.	3
Polenta	3	Add to boiling water, simmer for 20 minutes, remove from heat, cover, and let stand for several minutes before serving.	4
Quinoa	2	Rinse in fine mesh colander or flour sifter. Bring to a boil, cover, and simmer for 15 minutes.	3
Rye berries	3-4	Bring to a boil, cover, and simmer for 60 minutes.	3

Grain (1 cup dry)	Water or broth in cups	Cooking time/ special instructions	Yield in cups
Sorghum	3	Bring to boil, cover, reduce heat and simmer until tender, 50-60 minutes. Drain excess liquid.	3½
Spelt	3-4	Bring to boil and simmer until tender, 40-50 minutes. Drain excess liquid.	2½
Teff	3	Bring to a boil, cover, and simmer for 15-20 minutes.	2½
Wheat berries	3	Bring to a boil, cover, and simmer for 1.5-2 hours.	2½
Wild rice	2½	Bring to a boil, cover, and simmer for 40-45 minutes.	3

Sources: [116,117,114,119,120,121,122]

There are so many tasty ways to explore whole grains. Check out new ways to eat them at MelissasHealthyLiving.com and SuperKidsNutrition.com and aim to try a new one each month.

Ten tasty ways to boost whole grains

1. Experiment with quinoa. Quinoa makes a great substitute in fried rice, rice and beans, and rice bowls. As we mentioned before, brown rice can be a tasty and healthy part of your diet – just stick to the recommended weekly amount.[104,123]

2. For a twist to the classic hash browns breakfast, try making quinoa cakes or pinto bean mini burgers instead. Mix in some egg whites, green onion, herbs, and spices for added flavor.

3. In the mood for popcorn? Use it as salad croutons or add herbs and spices and use it as the whole grain in your meal. There are also countless ways to eat it as a flavorful snack!

4. Instead of your morning oatmeal, make breakfast porridge with a different whole grain. Amaranth breakfast porridge has a lovely, nutty flavor with a chewy texture. Ground buckwheat groats also serve as a good base for your creamy bowl.

5. Add some buckwheat into your soup. It also makes a great substitute for minestrone.

6. Look for puffed cereal, such as puffed Kamut, rice, millet, corn, or barley. These make for a quick and tasty breakfast and typically have no added sugar (but double check the label!). Try mixing any of them with some low-fat or fat-free Greek yogurt, your choice of milk, fresh or dried fruit, and a small handful of nuts or seeds.

7. Swap out some of the white/all-purpose flour in your recipes for whole grain flour. Start with ⅓ of your substitute and increase the ratio as desired. There are many whole grain/wheat-free flour alternatives, so you'll have plenty to choose from!

8. Mix a whole grain into your salads and stir-fries for added protein and flavor.

9. Make your own energy bars or granola. For the energy bars, mix rolled oats with your choice of the following: chopped nuts, nut butter, seeds, mashed banana, agave syrup or honey, and dried fruit. Bake on a cookie sheet at 350°F for about 20 minutes, or until firm. These make a great snack when you're on the go!

10. Does your dish call for noodles? Try using a whole grain version like buckwheat, spelt, or a quinoa-brown rice mix.

Legumes

Legumes, like milk, are classified as both carbohydrate and protein and play a dual role on your plate. They are considered a class of vegetable that provides carbohydrates and protein as well as fiber, vitamins, and minerals. Legumes include various types of beans, lentils, peas, and peanuts. A small ½ cup portion of cooked beans provides roughly 7 grams of protein and about 15 grams of carbohydrates. For vegan athletes, legumes (including soy!) are great sources of plant-based protein to incorporate into meals. Vegetarians can include these, along with dairy and eggs, as major protein sources. Omnivores can cut meat dishes in half by adding in beans or lentils to boost vitamins, minerals, fiber, and phytochemicals all while lowering food costs. Peanuts add a flavor boost to stir-fry dishes, salads and breakfast cereals and peas make a delicious addition to dips.

Legumes and pulses are a planet-friendly source of protein. Unlike other plant-foods, they are able to use atmospheric nitrogen as a source of plant nutrients. Because of this they require fewer nutrients from the soil and release significantly lower greenhouse gases compared to other crops. Utilizing lentils in crop rotations may positively influence the nitrogen content of the soil. Get some tasty lentil and legume recipes that fly solo or are accompanied by animal protein in the companion recipe book.[124,125]

Here are some examples of legumes, accompanied by their protein and carbohydrate (including fiber) content. All values are based on a 1-cup serving of cooked beans.

2.6 - Cooked Legume Content for a 1-cup Serving			
Legumes	Protein (g)	Carb (g)	Fiber (g)
Lentils	18	40	16
Edamame (soybeans), shelled	18	14	8
Navy beans (white)	16	46	19
Garbanzo beans	15	45	13
Kidney beans	15	40	13
Pinto beans	15	45	15
Black beans	15	41	15
Green peas	9	25	9

Peanuts aren't listed above because the serving size is 1 ounce, which provides around 7 grams protein, 5 grams of carbohydrate and 2 grams of fiber.

Different beans offer a variety of textures, flavors, and consistency. Make it a goal this month to discover your favorites!

COOKING TIP

If you don't eat beans regularly, start slowly! Beans contain a type of carbohydrate called oligosaccharide. Although oligosaccharides offer prebiotic benefits, they can cause gas. Luckily, oligosaccharides dissolve in water. If you cook beans yourself, soak them in the fridge overnight and drain the water. This removes some of the gas-causing oligosaccharides to help reduce gas while keeping some for a healthy gut. If you buy canned beans, rinse off their canning liquid.

Proper legume preparation

If the thought of cooking your own beans or lentils scares you, you've landed on the right page! You don't have to buy uncooked versions of either one. Both beans and lentils can be purchased pre-cooked in cans or in vacuum-sealed packaging. You can then get creative and puree your beans to boost the thickness of soups or make a tasty base for dips and sauces or use them to boost fiber and nutrition in mashed potatoes and brownies. Legumes are also a simple addition that you can toss into salads or whole grain bowls. Check out more ways to enjoy beans in our companion recipe book.

NUTRITION TIP

When buying pre-cooked or canned beans, look for low sodium or sodium-free on the package! Rinsing them in a colander can also lower sodium content by up to 40%.

Bean pasta as a source of protein

Regular white pasta is a great source of pre-race carbohydrates for endurance athletes and likely wins the spotlight at your average pasta dinner. Alternatively, grain-free pasta is quickly growing in popularity and availability – and for good reason! This type of pasta is an excellent choice when it comes to training meals because it provides athletes with both carbohydrate and protein for fuel. Plant-based proteins are key ingredients in a range of newly developed pasta varieties. Their main ingredients include lentils, chickpeas, almonds, soybeans, buckwheat, quinoa, spelt, or black beans. In addition to protein and carbohydrates, these types of pastas also deliver key vitamins, minerals, fiber, and phytonutrients.

Start with a small amount of bean pasta mixed in with your typical pasta. Some people love bean pasta right off the bat! Others may need to acclimate to the taste difference in bean pasta and experiment with cooking times that give you the preferred texture. Just like any high-fiber choice, give your gastrointestinal system time to adjust to bean pasta. If you're not used to them, a big bowl of bean pasta before your training session can leave you running to find a bathroom instead of running laps! Just like practicing for competition day, you should practice eating certain foods before any big event.

Lentil pasta is very high in fiber, and you need to determine if you can tolerate a full bowl – so start small! If you tend to have gas, you can always try a supplement with alpha-galactosidase, which is an enzyme that breaks down the oligosaccharides (the multiple carbohydrate branch) and should help decrease your symptoms. Make note that some bean enzyme supplements contain mannitol, a sugar alcohol which can actually cause gas for some people.

Here are some examples of different types of pasta based on a dry, 2-ounce serving, which yields roughly 1 cup of cooked pasta.[126] Garbanzo and lentil pasta typically have better taste acceptance than black bean pasta. Those with added tapioca mimic the traditional pasta taste more closely. Cooking bean pasta "al dente" improves the taste and texture, so you may want to cook it a minute less than instructed on the box. Here are some common bean pastas and the wonderful nutrient profiles they provide. We've also included some alternative grain pasta so you have them all in one place. For reference and for comparison purposes, your typical 2-ounce serving of refined pasta provides 7.5 grams protein, 43 grams carbohydrate, and 2 grams fiber.

2.7 - Types of Pastas – Values for a 2-ounce Serving			
Pasta	Protein (g)	Carb (g)	Fiber (g)
Legume pasta			
Green lentil	14	35	7
Red lentil	12	34	11
Black bean	13	28	9
Chickpea/garbanzo	13	33	7
Mixed grains/legumes pasta			
Lentil & quinoa	14	35	7
Black bean, brown rice, quinoa	12	35	7
Multi-grains/alternative grains pasta			
Kamut & quinoa	8	40	5
Kamut	10	40	6
Kamut & buckwheat	9	39	5
Spelt & buckwheat	6	41	4

Sources: [62,127, 128, 129, 130 ,131,132]

Don't forget that eating a variety of foods is crucial to helping the body get all the nutrients it needs to not only *survive* but to also *thrive*. Whole foods (including plant-based proteins) can provide athletes with the appropriate nutrition to perform at their highest levels. Ultimately, each individual should make the dietary decision that he or she feels is best for his or her body and lifestyle. Athletes should keep in mind that even though animal foods provide the highest amount of protein, it is indeed possible, when done correctly, to perform at an optimal level while relying heavily on plant-based foods.

Nut, Grain, and Root-Based Flours

Plant flours can also provide a healthy source of carbohydrate with some having higher amounts of protein than others. When baking, you'll often see nut, bean or root flours used in combination with whole wheat, brown rice, or another grain flour. Almond flour is amazing in cookies and works well combined with oat flour. Chickpea flour adds a unique flavor and dense quality to your baked goods and tastes great as flatbread. To start, you can try mixing chickpea flour and grain flour in your favorite baked treats. Substitute between 10-20% of the grain flour with chickpea flour, see how you like it, and increase from there. Each recipe is different, and sometimes it can take a few tries to perfect the ratio of flours. This doesn't mean that the first try is a waste. Think of it as a step in the right direction. You can try this with many of the other flours below too. It's time to get experimenting! Plant-based flours also mix well with mashed beans, avocado, and sweet potatoes. For example, our companion recipe book has a maple cocoa chickpea flour sweet potato brownie, that is delicious.

NUTRITION TIP

You have likely heard a lot about wheat (or more specifically, gluten) being the devil. Keep in mind that wheat has so many benefits for people who don't have Celiac disease or gluten-related symptoms. As you'll see below, it has 4 grams of protein per ¼ cup – a great way to boost more plant-based protein in your meals!

2.8 - Nutrient Composition of Plant-Based Flours for ¼-cup				
Flour type	Protein (g)	Carb (g)	Fat (g)	Fiber (g)
Almond	6	6	14	3
Coconut*	6	18	3	10
Garbanzo bean	5.5	13.5	1.5	2.5
Whole wheat	4	22	2	3
Buckwheat	4	21	1	3
Oat	4	17	2.5	1.5
Brown rice	3	30	1	2
Tiger nut	2	19	7	10
Cassava*	0	31	0	2

Source: USDA Food Composition Database[62] unless otherwise indicated by asterisk

*Bob's Red Mill's Nutrition Labels[133]

NUTRITION TIP

Cost Savings of Plant-Based Protein

Another benefit of focusing on plant-based protein sources is that it can help cut costs at the grocery store. Beans, legumes, tofu, and whole grains tend to be inexpensive staples compared to meat. This doesn't mean that you have to go completely vegetarian and eliminate animal proteins. Try to use the more expensive animal proteins as an accent rather than as the central ingredient in your meals to stretch your dollar. Shifting your focus to colorful vegetables and plant proteins will save you money and has numerous body benefits!

Melissa Halas MA, RDN, CDE

2.9 – Cost Comparison of Popular Protein-Rich Foods	
Food (average price)	Price per lb.
Pinto beans, dry, cooked[134]	$1.09
Black beans, dry, cooked[134]	$1.40
Chickpea pasta[135]	$5.40
Tofu[136]	$2.61
Salmon, wild Atlantic[137]	$7.99
Turkey breast[62,138,139]	$5.51
Turkey, ground, 93% lean[140]	$5.00
Chicken breast[141]	$3.49
Chicken, ground[142]	$3.99
Beef, ground[62,143]	$5.99
Beef, flank steak[144]	$8.99

A Look into Lectins

Lectins are proteins found in the outer shell of whole grains, pulses, and soybeans, and can also be found in fruits, vegetables, herbs, and spices. They are considered carbohydrate-binding proteins, and they serve as the protective coatings for the raw plant. Lectins can interact with human intestinal tracts and inhibit nutrient absorption.[145] Recently in the blogosphere, plant foods with lectin have been demonized. However, the studies cited are often performed in vitro (meaning not in humans!) with extracted lectin derivatives or in amounts that would never be reached in someone's diet.[146] Human bodies are so complex, and we can't assume that isolated, lab-derived experiments would yield identical reactions in the human body. The only well-documented dangers of lectin ingestion were observed in humans who consumed large amounts of raw or undercooked beans.[147] Given that raw beans are unappetizing and would be mechanically challenging to consume, we don't really have to worry much about this. A recent study in 2016 found that mushrooms, which contain lectins, have a potential anti-cancer effect.[148] This is why it's essential not to fall for food myths circulating online. Don't miss out on nutrients and their health benefits due to false claims.

Normal cooking processes for lectin-containing foods cause their lectin levels to plummet by 94-100%, making them perfectly safe for consumption. Soaking the foods prior to cooking only showed a modest decrease in lectins, but this trick may be beneficial in speeding up the cooking process.[149] Purchasing canned beans instead of cooking your own is an easy way to ensure your foods have been cooked thoroughly. The robust body of literature that supports whole grain, legume, and fruit and vegetable consumption for optimal health cannot be discredited by a handful of studies with partially faulty data. Including a variety of whole grains, cooked beans, peas, nuts, seeds and soybeans in your diet is both safe and encouraged to ensure you achieve adequate fiber and protein intake.[150]

NUTRITION TIP

Beware of fads or trending unsubstantiated nutrition claims – this is another reason to get your nutrition science from a trusted source, dietitian or nutrition scientist for expert guidance!

What Is Fiber?

Fiber is the indigestible part of plants that we eat. It works like a sponge to keep our digestive tracts clean and contributes to lowering serum cholesterol and warding off certain cancers.[27] Fiber has numerous benefits for good health and disease prevention, including lowering the risk of heart disease, managing type 2 diabetes, helping with weight loss, promoting healthy bowel movements, and decreasing inflammation and osteoarthritis. There are two main forms of fiber – insoluble and soluble. Resistant starch is also referred to as non-digestible carbohydrates or fiber, but it's not a primary source of fiber.

Insoluble Fiber

- Foods high in insoluble fiber include fruits and vegetables, wheat bran, and whole grains.
- Insoluble fiber speeds up transit time, increases fecal volume, and increases the number of stools.[151] This type of fiber is beneficial when constipation occurs.
- You can think of insoluble fiber as the rough part of a sponge since it "scrapes" and "cleans" the sides of the digestive tract.

Soluble Fiber

- Foods high in soluble fiber include legumes, lentils, oats, seeds, nuts, peas, and certain vegetables, such as squash and carrots.[152]
- Soluble fiber slows down transit time, draws water into the digestive tract, binds to nutrients in the intestines, and decreases their absorption.[152] Some good nutrients are lost, but the current fiber recommendations below account for this. Soluble fiber is good for both diarrhea and constipation by creating a more "regular" frequency of bowel movements.
- Soluble fiber is especially important in lowering excess cholesterol, as it binds to cholesterol and eliminates it through the feces. You can think of soluble fiber as the soft part of a sponge soaking up the fluids, and just like a sponge, it helps you clean up a spill.

While insoluble and soluble fibers have different actions, both types are needed in a healthy diet. The U.S. Dietary Guidelines recommend 25 grams of fiber per day for women (19-50 years old) and 38 grams of fiber per day for men (19-50 years old). This should be in combination with drinking plenty of fluids to support a healthy and regularly functioning digestive tract. For women over 50 years old, the recommendation is 21 grams of fiber per day, and for men over 50 years old, it is 30 grams of fiber per day.[153]

If you're not accustomed to eating complex (high-fiber) carbohydrates you should consider gradually adding them into your diet in order to allow your body to slowly adjust to the fiber content of these foods. Eating higher fiber foods at regular meals (when carbohydrate loading isn't needed) can give the body the opportunity to grow accustomed to fiber. Many people experience stomach distress when they eat high-fiber foods immediately before training/competing. This happens because the fiber holds onto water in the gut, causes bloating, and slows down digestion. Some athletes have a tough stomach and can tolerate higher fiber foods before exercising, but this can vary from person to person; and remember, what works for one person might not work for the next. If you are unsure of how your body will respond, just like with carbohydrate loading, experiment with fibrous foods to see what sits well in your stomach and how much time you need for digestion before exercising. It often takes time to acclimate to higher fiber carbohydrates. Continue to try them in small amounts to allow your digestive tract time to adjust.[154]

Some people may notice they tolerate a higher volume of higher fiber meals and snacks better before lower intensity exercise than higher intensity exercise. Practice what works best for you! But remember, no new high-fiber foods (or new foods in general!) the day before or on competition day.

NUTRITION TIP

Lentils, although high in soluble fiber, have a tendency to speed up transit time and increase bowel movements in some individuals.

Steps to Slowly Increase Your Fiber Intake

Step 1 – Determine your fiber baseline

How many grams do you need? As you just read above, the recommendation is 25 grams per day for women and 38 grams per day for men. If you are over 50 years of age, the recommendations are 21 grams and 30 grams, respectively. Now that you know how much you need, how many grams do you normally consume per day? You can find this out by checking the Nutrition Facts labels on the foods you normally eat, or by using the UDSA Food Composition Database. This database has standard references for foods, as well as some branded products. Avoid publicly sourced data on other websites, as they typically have large margins of error.

Step 2 – Increase your fiber by focusing first on one food group per week

If your fiber intake is below the recommendation for your age and gender, your digestive health and overall health will most likely benefit from increasing your fiber intake. However, if your body is not used to it, eating a lot of fiber in one meal or in one day can cause uncomfortable side effects, like diarrhea and bloating.

To prevent these side effects, try gradually increasing your fiber intake by changing one thing each week. Here are a few ideas to try:

- Add a serving of vegetables to your breakfast, like heating up frozen peppers and cooking them with your eggs.
- Swap out your traditional pasta for buckwheat or use half garbanzo bean pasta.

Melissa Halas MA, RDN, CDE

- Add half an avocado to a meal like a sandwich or salad.
- Make the switch from wheat or white bread to 100% whole wheat or whole grain.
- Make a grain or polenta the base for your burger in place of a bun.
- Add in cooked quinoa or barley and additional frozen vegetables to canned soups.
- Have a serving of raw vegetables or whole grain crackers with 2 tablespoons hummus, edamame dip, or Greek yogurt as a snack. See our companion recipe book for tasty mixes.
- Have a handful of nuts as a snack, or sprinkle them on oatmeal, yogurt, or salads.
- Eat fruit for dessert and top with granola, oatmeal, chia seeds, nuts or amaranth porridge with a drizzle of honey and dash of cinnamon.

Step 3 – Simultaneously with Step 2, increase your fluid intake

Fiber pulls water from your body into your intestines so that it can pass through smoothly. So, while increasing fiber too quickly can cause diarrhea, it can also cause constipation if you're not drinking enough water or other fluid. This should remind you of the protein fact we discussed earlier as well. When increasing fluid intake, remember to choose unsweetened beverages. Don't forget that there are many foods that are high in water that are also high in fiber such as fruits and vegetables.

Step 4 – Consider the timing of high-fiber meals

If you're going for a run in the morning, the day before your run, have a high-fiber meal for lunch, not dinner. If you have it for dinner, you may end up having to find a restroom during your run.

Carbohydrate Needs For Athletes

General Carbohydrate Needs

When we went over the carbohydrate basics, we mentioned that glycogen is stored in the liver and the muscles. Remember that a diet higher in plant-based foods typically increases glycogen storage. Now we're going to dive into how you can maximize your stores and make sure you're fueling properly for any exercise that you're going to do.

The first step in assessing the proper approach for carbohydrate loading is to understand typical carbohydrate needs. These typical carbohydrate needs for athletes range from 3-12 grams of carbohydrate per kilogram of body weight per day depending on the intensity of activity as noted below, with more intense and time-consuming training requiring more.[155]

2.10 - Intensity Classifications for Carbohydrate Needs[156]

- **Light** – minimal changes in breathing
- **Moderate** – noticeably faster heart rate than at rest, requires moderate effort
- **High/Very High** – large increase in heart rate, faster and more labored breathing, requires a lot of effort to perform

	Activity	Amount of carb	Grams of carb/day for a 140 lb. (63.6 kg) person	Grams of carb/day for a 180 lb. (81.8 kg) person
Light	Skill-based/low Intensity	3-5 g/kg/day	191-318	245-409
Moderate	1 hour/day	5-7 g/kg/day	318-445	409-573
High	1-3 hours/day	6-10 g/kg/day	382-636	491-818
Very high	4-5 hours/day	8-12 g/kg/day	509-763	654-982

2.11 - Example of Carbohydrate Servings[65]

~15 grams of carbohydrate

Honey, fruit, starchy vegetables, legumes, and whole grains

- 1 tablespoon honey
- ½ cup frozen mango
- 1 cup blackberries
- ½ cup unsweetened apple sauce
- 1 Medjool date
- ½ cup orange juice
- 2 tablespoons raisins
- ½ whole grain English muffin
- 1 piece sprouted whole grain bread
- ½ cup shredded wheat

- ½ cup cooked oatmeal
- 1 large, round, brown rice cake
- ⅓ cup cooked whole wheat pasta
- ⅓ cup cooked brown basmati rice
- ½ cup cooked bean pasta rotini, like chickpea
- ⅓ tablespoons cooked black beans
- ⅓ cup lentils
- ½ cup boiled potato
- 2½ cups popcorn

2.12 - Example of Carbohydrate Servings[65]
Dairy
• 1 cup of milk: 12 grams • 8 ounces nonfat plain Greek yogurt: 9 grams • 1 cup cottage cheese: 8 grams

Carbohydrates provide immediate fuel but are also stored so they can be utilized for exercise. Our bodies are able to store 300-400 grams of carbohydrate as glycogen in our muscles and 75-100 grams in our liver.[80] The blood only holds about 5 grams of glucose. Blood glucose is tightly regulated to make sure we have enough glucose readily available for our bodies and brain to function properly. When blood glucose and muscle and liver glycogen stores have been depleted, the body utilizes other sources of energy to create glucose. This may lead to the breakdown of muscle into free amino acids that are turned into glucose. Conserving muscle power and reserves is essential for all athletes' performance – another reason why adequate and proper intake of carbohydrate is needed. Sufficient carbohydrate intake should also be a top priority when you're focused on fueling.

NUTRITION TIP

The 60-90-minute exercise threshold for when you have gone through your glycogen stores and need supplemental carbohydrate is an important one to remember, especially for those of you who are endurance athletes.

Even recreational athletes or fitness enthusiasts who are going for a long bike ride or hiking for longer than an hour will most likely need a carbohydrate snack to maximize endurance and reduce fatigue after exercise.

Best Choice Carbohydrates with Sport

While your food choices day to day should primarily focus on complex carbs, there is a certain time and place for the more easily digestible carbs. These fast-acting carbs can actually be beneficial *before*, *during* and *after* activity so that your body can take up the glucose quickly and use it as fuel, or quickly replenish what was used after exercise. Other than this, you can go back to focusing on adding more complex, nutrient-dense carbohydrates.

One of the main reasons for this emphasis on simple carbohydrates is that prior to a long training session, race, or during an event, you need to replete carbohydrates quickly. Complex carbs contain more fiber or bulk, which can lead to emergency bathroom issues or stomach discomfort. Gels or energy electrolyte drinks are quick and simple solutions if your gut has trouble with more bulky foods prior to or during exercise. We'll dive more into these later. As with anything else, always try these out during practice or training sessions if it's your first time experimenting – never on race day!

There are now also certain products that have slow-acting carbohydrates that are typically made of hydrolyzed cornstarch. They are easier on the stomach and help elongate carbohydrate digestion for more sustained energy throughout the workout.

These types of products are usually consumed shortly before endurance exercise, and depending on the event, might be supplemented with another sports product during exercise (i.e., gel, chew, sports drink). Unfortunately, these products are usually quite costly, so a simple and effective alternative is to consume a combination of carbohydrate and low protein instead before you get going on an endurance activity. If you only have about an hour for digestion, think about a pea protein smoothie with pomegranate juice and a banana with low-fat Greek yogurt. Keep in mind that for endurance activities you'll still want to pack some quick acting carbohydrates like apple juice, graham crackers, fig bars, 2-3 dates, dried banana, or honey chews. You just want to make sure you don't overdo it on the protein because this can decrease transit time and lead to stomach discomfort for some people.

Carbohydrates as Glycogen

Remember that glycogen is the storage form of glucose stored primarily in the liver and muscles? When glucose is not readily available, glycogen is broken down to provide needed fuel. Muscle glycogen is the major source of energy and most easily accessible during exercise. If you're not replenishing those depleted glycogen stores, you'll have to tap into liver glycogen. Liver glycogen can be turned into glucose and transported through the blood and to muscles when needed. But don't go there! Refuel to maximize performance.

Similarly, liver glycogen can travel to the brain and other organs that need energy if blood glucose is not immediately available. It is important to note that glycogen stored in the muscle can only be used by that muscle tissue. Liver glycogen is willing to share with the rest of the body. Yay, liver! Therefore, if an athlete were to be on a low-carbohydrate diet, they could potentially be running out of energy due to the low amount of stored glycogen in their muscles and depleted liver glycogen.

Glycogen is usually depleted over a 24-hour period. This demonstrates the importance of carbohydrates for all athletes in order to replenish stores, regardless of whether they practice endurance or strength-based sports. Regular intake of carbohydrates at meals, snacks, or when refueling during exercise helps ensure you always have something stored in your glycogen tank when you need a boost of energy.[157,158]

Carbohydrate Loading

Carbohydrate/Glycogen Loading Basics

With a better understanding of the body's use of glucose and glycogen, carbohydrate loading should hopefully be a bit easier to tackle. Carbohydrate loading is a practice often used by endurance athletes before a competition because it temporarily increases glycogen stores. You want to make sure your tank is full when it comes time for the competition! It is a widely known and utilized practice because depleted glycogen stores can lead to a decrease in energy and a decline in performance.[159] You've heard, "eat a pasta dinner the night before a big race." This is based on the concept of carbohydrate loading. However, over the past several decades, the recommendations for timing and amount of carbohydrate loading have changed due to some new findings of how the body holds onto and uses glycogen. To figure out if you really need to buy into this carb loading trick, use the simplified tips below as a guide.

Glycogen Supercompensation

Carbohydrate loading, also known as glycogen loading or glycogen supercompensation, has been practiced with different approaches over the years. The purpose as mentioned before is to attempt to delay the onset of fatigue. Glycogen supercompensation was initially comprised of a 3-day carbohydrate depletion (low carbohydrate diet) with normal training, followed by a 3-day exercise taper with carbohydrate loading – a total of ~6-7 days.[160] With this approach, glycogen levels weren't just topping off the tanks, they went beyond the normal concentrations of glycogen –hence, the term which has remained today, "supercompensation."[161]

Then research found the depletion phase was not necessary, resulting in a 3-day protocol for carbohydrate loading for endurance athletes. Now newer research shows that a 36- to 48-hour protocol of 10-12 grams of carbohydrate per kilogram of body weight per day can still maximize glycogen stores.[160] One of the biggest reasons for this change is that studies observed that extremely high levels of glycogen are broken down faster than moderately high levels. Overloading the body with glycogen past a certain point doesn't provide any additional performance benefit.

Remember the hydration fact that 3 grams of water are bound to each gram of stored glycogen? This is helpful to remember when carb loading. If your body stores an additional 300-400 grams of glycogen, along with 900-1,200 grams of water, your body weight will increase about 1,200-1,600 grams or 2.5-3.5 pounds above your normal training weight during the loading phase. Getting a feel for this before the competition is to your advantage!

WHO SHOULD CARB LOAD?

- Anyone exercising for endurance events greater than 90 minutes.
- Long-distance runners, swimmers, bicyclists, triathletes, cross-country skiers, and similar athletes.
- Athletes who are involved in prolonged stop-and-go activities, such as soccer, lacrosse, and tournament-play sports like tennis and handball. This depends on the position played and the duration.

This is not for long training sessions. Athletes already meet their needs with the recommended carbohydrate per kilogram of body weight per day.

Impacts of Fitness on Carb Loading

Speaking of fitness, the level of training and fitness comes into play in other ways as well. Research has also found that more trained individuals take less time to load than less trained individuals.[57] No one needs to carbohydrate load for a typical day of training at the gym. This could just lead to overeating or feeling bloated, and all the extra calories can contribute to unnecessary weight gain! Instead, a focus on getting enough quality carbohydrates at meals, snacks, and refueling right during training – not consuming excess – is key.

Some recreational athletes like to train and participate occasionally in intense events, like bikeathons, marathons, or triathlons. In these situations, carbohydrate loading is a strategy that can help performance. If this doesn't apply to you then skip to the carbohydrate timing section. If it does apply, read on to "So How Can Athletes Carbohydrate Load Correctly?"

So How Can Athletes Carbohydrate Load Correctly?

If you've identified yourself as an athlete who can benefit from a carb load protocol, keep reading. Carbohydrate loading occurs through the accumulation of muscle glycogen through a large dietary intake of carbohydrates for a few days prior to exercise, along with a corresponding decrease in activity.[162] Ideally, carbohydrate loading takes place 2-3 days before a competition; however, similar results may also be obtained within one day for a shorter competition.[18,80]

How to Carbohydrate Load

In order to get the most out of carbohydrate loading, the athlete must be endurance trained in their sport.[77] Carbohydrate loading would entail 10-12 grams of carbohydrate per kilogram of body weight for the 36-48 hours leading up to the race, tournament, or competition.[163] This can help athletes keep both muscle and liver glycogen levels intact while ensuring sufficient glucose is in their blood during exercise.[78,159] This is further shown in the carbohydrate overview chart at the end of this chapter.

A key factor with carbohydrate loading to note is that your total calories consumed are not changing.[84] Instead, the increase in carbohydrates should be replacing the calories from fat and some protein during this time frame. You will be decreasing bulk and helping to prevent gastrointestinal distress during your exercise.[163]

Additionally, some athletes may have problems tolerating the high-fiber intake that comes along with carbohydrate loading. To mitigate this potential problem, as with anything that has to do with nutrition and exercise, practice to see what works. Implementing a test carb loading session for a long training session or a lower priority practice race can help identify pitfalls and reduce troublesome symptoms. As mentioned previously, some athletes can help decrease gastrointestinal distress by focusing on eating lower fiber foods such as pasta, white rice, cereals, sports bars, and gels in the final two days.[18,80]

With all of this in mind, this is not the time to be eating plate upon plate of lentil pasta! You can still include some lower fiber, plant-based proteins, as tolerated. By practicing a carbohydrate loading technique, including which foods to consume and what you can tolerate, you will be better prepared for the big race or event when it really counts!

HIGH FRUCTOSE FOODS

Overconsumption of high fructose foods may be a trigger for stomach discomfort, so it is another factor to account for in optimizing pre-competition nutrition. Some high fructose foods include honey, raisins, apple sauce, dried or fresh figs, dried prunes, boysenberries, cherries, pears, mangos, watermelon, tamarillos, apple juice, and grape juice.[62,164] These foods are tolerated by most people and athletes; however, you may not want to consume high amounts of these when carb loading.

Can You Load from Whole Grains?

Loading from only whole grains may make it difficult to reach the recommended daily amounts of carbohydrates in those last couple of days before an event. This is why a low-residue diet (think low-fiber) is recommended for athletes who are going to participate in longer events. It is also important to note that if you don't normally consume whole grains on a daily basis, consuming whole grains in large quantities in the days leading up to the competition is counterproductive. Whole grains are high in fiber and a body that is not used to them may experience overload, leading to constipation, gas, or loose stools on game day, as mentioned previously. Runners may experience abdominal discomfort and urgency to move their bowels while running. Someone who is used to eating mostly whole grains may tolerate whole grain loading better, but will still need some refined grains. Everyone is different and what works for one person, may not work for another person. Again, fueling strategies and food options should be tested before the big game or race.

Carbohydrate Timing

A Look at Pre-Exercise Carbohydrate Timing

The amount of carbohydrate you should eat depends on the amount of time you have before you exercise. Here is a simple chart to follow in terms of quantity of carbohydrate:

2.13 - Pre-Exercise Carbohydrate Timing			
Amount of time before exercise	Carbohydrate to consume	Carbohydrate for a 140 lb. (63.6kg) person	Carbohydrate for a 180 lb. (81.8kg) person
1 hour	1 g/kg	64 g	81 g
2 hours	2 g/kg	127 g	164 g
3 hours	3 g/kg	191 g	245 g
4 hours	4 g/kg	254 g	327 g

For any time less than an hour before exercise, consuming an easily digestible (think low-fiber) form of carbohydrate of about 30 grams can be beneficial for your performance.[80]

Here is an example of how the timing would work around exercise/ competition at different times of the day:

- Morning events: eat low-fiber, low-fat, moderate protein breakfast; consume adequate fluids, and have a small carbohydrate-rich snack after warm-up[163]
    - Restore liver glycogen after an overnight fast and ensure your body is properly hydrated.
- Early- to mid-afternoon events: eat a substantial breakfast and a pre-competition meal for lunch
- Late afternoon events: eat breakfast, lunch, and snacks
- Evening events: eat breakfast, lunch, and a pre-competition meal for dinner[78]

2.14 - Carbohydrates During Endurance Exercise			
Length of exercise	**Amount of carb needed**	**Type of carb**	**Examples**
<45 minutes	None		
45-75 minutes	Small amounts and/or mouth rinse	Glucose or maltodextrin	Glucose or maltodextrin rinse
1-2.5 hours	30-60 g/hour	Glucose or a mix	Sports hydration mix, gels
>2.5-3 hours	Up to 90 g/hour	Must be from multiple transportable carbohydrates (i.e., glucose + fructose)	Chews, gels (read ingredients)

Adapted from ACSM Position Stand[78]

If you look at the 45-75-minute time frame, you'll notice that small amounts and/or mouth rinsing is recommended. Mouth rinsing is a process of swishing a mouthful of a carbohydrate solution in your mouth (swish and expel or drink), which stimulates brain regions that are involved in motor control, reward, and perception of fatigue. This can lead to increased work output and enhanced mood.[78]

You may also notice that for athletes doing ultra-endurance exercise greater than 2.5-3 hours, multiple transportable carbohydrates are needed. This is because your glucose transporter (SGLT1) in your intestines can only absorb 60 grams per hour. So, to get around the 60-gram limit and take in even more carbohydrates to fuel, find a product or food combination that has both glucose and fructose and work up to the 90 grams per hour. This works because fructose has its own transporter (GLUT5)!

Here are a few common items used to meet those needs:
- sports drinks (14-18 grams carbohydrates per 8 ounces)
- sports gels (20-30 grams carbohydrates per gel)
- sports bars (19-50 grams carbohydrates per bar)

Post Workout: Refueling Best

Equally important to consuming carbohydrates after a workout is making sure that the body is being refueled with the proper amount of protein. Consuming sufficient protein following exercise helps athletes prevent delayed onset muscle soreness and is associated with a subsequent workout that is performed at a higher intensity.[165] Remember that a minimum of 1.2-1.7 grams of protein per kilogram of body weight per day is needed to allow for tissue synthesis and repair in most endurance athletes. We also discussed that some athletes in sports that require more muscle mass (weightlifting, football) may require closer to a daily intake of 2 grams of protein per kilogram of body weight per day.[166] However, most exercise enthusiasts, even those trying to gain muscle, don't need this much protein. Competitive bodybuilders can require as much as 3 grams of protein per kilogram of lean body mass, and sometimes even more than this.[167]

PROTEIN TIP

Protein should be consumed throughout the day at each meal, and at times directly following exercise when possible. Consume 0.25-0.3 grams of protein per kilogram of body weight, as it helps muscles rebuild and recover.[78,167] For a 140-pound person, this is 16 grams of protein, and for a 185-pound person this is 21 grams of protein. This is why you'll typically see a range of 15-25 grams of protein to aim for post-exercise. Separating your intake throughout the day helps you meet your overall needs.

Pairing up carbohydrates and protein

Once you're done with exercise, replenishing the glycogen that was used and repairing the small micro-tears in your muscles is key for proper recovery.

Consumption of a recovery meal is optimal after an intense workout for serious athletes. If increasing your muscle mass is a goal, even exercise enthusiasts should be aiming for a post-workout snack or meal. The key is to maximize the amount of carbohydrates and protein your body is absorbing and using after exercise. The body has an enhanced ability to use the carbohydrates and protein directly after exercise to replenish muscle glycogen stores and to maximize muscle protein synthesis. However, the exact window hasn't been identified. Previously, sports dietitians recommended eating a combination of carbohydrate and protein within 90 minutes of training in addition to regular protein throughout the day. More recent research shows now that focusing on reaching total protein needs in a day, and aiming to eat every 3-4 hours can still help reach your goals. Therefore, aim to consume a meal or snack within 3-4 hours of exercise. If you have another session later in the day or have specific body composition goals, you may need to focus on more immediate food intake.[78] If you're not getting the results you want, try eating within a shorter window and including leucine sources.

With this timing in mind, it is likely that the time post-exercise falls is within 3-4 hours after an athlete has eaten last. This is why aiming to have a snack or meal after exercise is typically recommended. If your schedule does not allow for a full sit-down meal after exercise, combining your post-workout protein with a carbohydrate source in the form of a healthy snack following exercise can allow for accelerated muscle building, repair, and restoration of energy stores. In general, you'll be aiming for 1.0-1.2 grams of carbohydrate per kilogram of body weight and 0.25-0.3 grams of protein per kilogram of body weight in this meal or snack.[78]

For active individuals that wouldn't classify themselves as serious athletes or as someone who is going through hard training, it is best to keep track of the timing of meals, and how you feel after exercise. If you're shaky from hunger and your stomach is growling, a snack or meal is indicated. However, for those with a history of being overweight or monitoring their weight, adding a snack could lead to weight gain. A balanced recovery meal at your normal eating time is a simple approach and goal to follow.

Two-a-day training

Those who participate in a two-a-day training schedule should consume sufficient protein and carbohydrate after their first session to assist in recovery and help improve performance in the next training session. It is recommended to consume 1.0-1.2 grams of carbohydrate per kilogram of body weight per hour for the 4 hours after your first workout to make sure you've replenished your glycogen stores.[78] Replenishing carbohydrate stores are key here so that you have the fuel to meet the demands of your second session. If you have the choice, two-a-day training sessions should be spread out for recovery, ideally 6-8 hours apart. Of course, this is not always possible, especially with collegiate athletes. Nutrition timing thus becomes that much more important!

Strength athletes

If you are competing in weights or lifting twice per day, it's best practice to be eating after each workout for recovery. This is due to the fact that you need to consume a certain amount of protein to maximize gains, and if you don't eat frequently enough, your body won't be able to absorb all of the protein that you need. Timing is key to make sure you're able to take in all of the calories needed for growth. It is not uncommon for these types of athletes, or even collegiate athletes, to consume 4-5 meals per day (or even more!) containing carbs and protein to ensure adequate calorie, carbohydrate, and protein intake for their needs and the demands of their sport.

Snacking techniques

Snacking is required for:
- Competitive athletes who have conditioning or practices twice a day.
- Physique athletes who are also doing High Intensity Interval Training (HIIT).
- Exercise enthusiasts who have specific body composition goals or are exercising twice a day (i.e. Biking in the morning and strength training in the evening).

What should be in the snack?
- The amount of carbohydrate and protein in this snack will vary significantly depending on your sport, goals, and time and composition of the next meal.
- Here's a general example: A snack with both protein and carbohydrate, such as a fruit smoothie with nut butter and seeds or a chickpea protein brownie (in our companion book).
- This is a great reason to meet with an RD and get more individualized guidance.

Why is snacking important?
- It can be beneficial for maintaining lean muscle mass, recovering from the first workout, and reducing muscle soreness following the second workout.
- It can help meet elevated protein needs, and ensure muscle protein synthesis will occur. It's difficult to meet protein needs at meals alone, or if met, too much would need to be consumed and inefficiently utilized.

2.15 - Snack Options with 20-30 Grams of Protein and 1-4 Servings of Carbohydrate

Snack options	Ingredients	Protein (g)	Carbs (g)
Bean & tomato salad	• 1½ cup white or black beans • ¼ cup chopped tomatoes • 1 tsp. balsamic vinegar • ½ tsp. liquid aminos or soy sauce • 1 tsp. olive oil • Italian seasoning to taste	22	63
Pea protein shake	• 2 scoops (or about 27g) pea protein[168] with 8 oz. water • 1 frozen banana, medium • Vanilla extract and cinnamon to taste	22	29
Edamame and pumpkin seed mix	• 1 cup salted edamame • 2 Tbsp. pumpkin seeds	21	18
Baked tofu with a side of blueberries	• 8 oz. baked tofu sticks[169] • 1 Tbsp. honey • 1 Tbsp. shredded fresh ginger • 1 Tbsp. balsamic vinegar • 1 Tbsp. soy dressing • ½ tsp. garlic powder • ¾ cup blueberries	23	44
Yogurt with cherries and chia seeds	• 1 cup plain nonfat Greek yogurt • ½ cup frozen cherries, defrosted • 1 Tbsp. chia seeds	22	32
Bread with peanut butter and a string cheese	• 1 slice of whole grain bread • 2 Tbsp. peanut butter • 2 sticks skim string cheese	22	23
Turkey & cheese roll-ups with apple slices	• 2 medium slices turkey breast (2 oz.) • 1 slice cheese • 1 medium apple, sliced	23	31
Lentil, feta, and tomato	• ¾ cup lentils • ⅓ cup feta • 2 thick slices tomato	21	34
Cottage cheese and strawberries	• 1 cup strawberries • ¾ cup cottage cheese	21	20

(See MelissasHealthyLiving.com for full recipes)

FOOD FEATURE: OATS

Want to substitute a light and airy gluten-free flour into your baked goods? Try blending oats in your blender or food processor until they reach a fluffy flour-like consistency. They lack gluten, so you need a binding agent. Try a chia "egg" for a fiber, omega-3s, and calcium boost.

OAT FACTS:
- Contain 11-15% protein by weight[62]
- Beta-glucan, a type of fiber in oats, has cholesterol and blood glucose lowering abilities.[170]
- One cup of cooked oats is a good source of polyphenols, which have antioxidant properties.[170] Polyphenols offer a powerhouse of body benefits, from reducing the risk of heart disease and certain types of cancer (including breast cancer) to helping protect against brain aging.[33]
- Oats are almost always found as a whole grain (with bran and endosperm), even in packaged goods.[171]
- One cup of cooked oats is a good source of magnesium.[62]
- A great option for Celiac or gluten-free diets - be sure to choose gluten-free oats

FIT TIP: Make no-bake oat bites for the week for an easy breakfast you can pack in your gym bag each morning for a post-workout treat!

Overview of Carbohydrates with Exercise

Now that we covered the ins and outs of carbohydrates around exercise, here is a summary table **(2.16 - Overview of Carbohydrates with Exercise on pages 94-95)** for reference whenever you want to fine-tune your fueling strategy.

2.16 - Overview of Carbohydrates with Exercise

Timing	Situation	Carbohydrate needs	Example carbohydrate regimen for a 154lb (70 kg) person	Additional tips
Fueling basics	Preparing for exercise <90 min	7-12 g/kg for 24 hours	490-840 g	Timing, type, and the amount should be individualized to event and athlete's tolerance
Carb loading	Preparing for exercise >90 min	10-12 g/kg/d for 36-48 hours	700-840 g for 36-48 hours	• Low fiber/residue • Small, regular snacks may be better tolerated • Timing, type, and the amount should be individualized to event and athlete's tolerance • Avoid high fat/fiber
Fueling pre-exercise	Before exercise >60 min long	1-4 g/kg consumed 1-4 hours before training	70-280 g consumed 1-4 hours before training	Timing, type, and the amount should be individualized to the event and athlete's tolerance
Fueling during exercise	<45 minutes	None		
	45-75 minutes	Small amounts and/or mouth rinse		Mouth rinse should be true carbohydrate (not artificial sweetener)

Melissa Halas MA, RDN, CDE

	1-2.5 hours	30-60 g/hour	
	>2.5-3 hours	Up to 90 g/hour	Multiple transportable carbohydrates
Refueling quickly	<8 hours of recovery between intense sessions	1-1.2 g/kg/hour for 1st 4 hours, then general fueling	

Sources: [78,84]

Part 3:
FATS

Where Does Fat Fit In?

N ADDITION TO PROTEIN AND carbohydrates, fats – also known as lipids – comprise the third macronutrient within the human diet. As with the other two macronutrients, athletes should be mindful of the types and amounts of fats they consume. While limiting certain types of fats should be a focus (to decrease the risk of cardiovascular disease, diabetes, and cancer), making sure you incorporate health-promoting fats is just as important. Including these healthy fats in your diet to create balanced meals can lead to improved health and enhanced athletic performance.[172] On the elemental level, fats are comprised of the same three elements as carbohydrates: carbon, oxygen, and hydrogen. There are three main types of fats:

- **Unsaturated fats**: the ones we love!
- **Saturated fats**: the ones we should limit to 10% or less of our daily energy
- **Trans fats**: the ones we should avoid

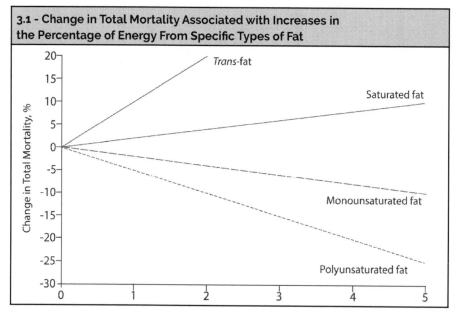

3.1 - Change in Total Mortality Associated with Increases in the Percentage of Energy From Specific Types of Fat

Source: JAMA Intern Med [173]

Functions of Fat in the Body

Fats have many valuable functions in our bodies that are important for overall health and maximizing exercise performance. They are needed for energy storage and production, storage and absorption of the fat-soluble vitamins (vitamins A, D, E, and K), and for cellular signaling and hormone production.[174] Fats also help insulate and protect our internal organs, provide cushioning, keep our brains healthy, contribute to immune system functioning, and reproduction in addition to other important metabolic roles.[175]

Another important role of fat in regards to exercise is for during prolonged exercise or exercise at a low to moderate intensity. At these exercise intensities, fat is the main fuel source. These "fat-burning" zones are highly variable between different individuals. However, trained athletes typically use more fat than untrained athletes at higher intensities.[163]

Fats to Focus on for Optimal Health and Performance

While fat contains 9 calories per gram, not all fats are created equal. Here's what you need to know about the different types.

Unsaturated Fats

For optimal heart, brain, and eye health focus on getting your fat from unsaturated sources. Unsaturated fats are found in foods such as nuts and nut butters, avocados, plant oils that are liquid at room temperature, seeds and seed butters, and fish.[176] There are two main categories of unsaturated fats –monounsaturated and polyunsaturated fats.

Monounsaturated fats

Monounsaturated fats have a chemical structure that contains one double bond. Additionally, monounsaturated fats are a source of vitamin E, an important antioxidant with cancer-preventing properties.[177,178] Good sources of monounsaturated fats include avocados, olive and canola oils, certain nuts such as almonds and pecans, and certain seeds such as sesame seeds and pumpkin seeds.[170,179]

Polyunsaturated fats

Polyunsaturated fats are fat molecules that contain two or more double bonds. Good sources of polyunsaturated fats include certain oils such as flaxseed, sunflower, and soybean oils, as well as walnuts, fish, and flax seeds. Canola oil also provides polyunsaturated fat.[179] If you don't want to include genetically modified organisms (GMOs) in your diet, choose organic or non-GMO canola oil, as it's typically a genetically modified food.

There are two main types of polyunsaturated fats: omega-3 and omega-6 fatty acids (omega-6s). Omega-6s are found in some vegetable oils, nuts, and seeds.[179] While the typical American diet generally contains an adequate amount of omega-6 fatty acids, omega-3s may be lacking.[180] In general, it is best to focus most on getting sufficient amounts of omega-3s in your diet. Here are a few of the basics you should know about omega-3s and how to get more of them.

Omega-3 and essential fatty acids

It is important to make sure you are getting enough polyunsaturated fats; specifically, certain omega-3s, which are especially important for athletes as they play a role in reducing inflammation and free radicals that can develop during exercise. In addition, they improve airway functioning and can act as a vasodilator.[176] Preliminary research shows that omega-3s may also help with muscle flexibility, better range of motion, and muscle recovery.[181-184] They also help maintain good heart health by lowering triglycerides and blood pressure and maintaining brain and eye health.

NUTRITION TIP

Boost omega-3 fatty acids in your diet to help lower inflammation. Aim for at least one plant-based serving of an omega-3-rich food per day, such as walnuts, flax meal, or chia seeds. If you're eating an animal source of omega-3s, include some plant-based too. For example, have a meal with salmon and crushed walnuts.

The three important types of omega-3s include alpha-linolenic acid (ALA), eicosapentaenoic acid (EPA), and docosahexaenoic acid (DHA). ALA *must* be consumed from food sources or supplements, as it cannot be made within the body. ALA can be converted to EPA, and EPA can be converted to DHA; however, these conversions are not the most efficient. The conversion from ALA to EPA has a rate of 5-15%, whereas less than 1% of ALA converts to DHA.[185] For vegetarians ALA is a good source of polyunsaturated fatty acids. Because of this, it is also important to ensure adequate intake of EPA and DHA from food or supplements.[186] Research has shown mixed results for the individual benefits of ALA. For those with high cholesterol levels, ALA has been shown to lower lipid levels, reduce vascular inflammation, and reduce blood pressure. There have also been documented benefits of ALA from canola oil, reducing the risk of coronary heart disease (CHD). Walnuts, the only tree nuts that are an excellent source of ALA, have shown numerous health benefits, including lowering the risk of CVD and stroke. Plant-sources of omega-3s have also been shown to have a protective effect on bone metabolism. However, the most cardioprotective effect is the consumption of ALA, EPA, and DHA in the diet.[180,187]

Food sources of ALA, EPA & DHA

ALA sources include some plant oils such as flaxseed, canola, and soybean oils. Chia seeds and walnuts are other good sources.[188] Chart 3.2 outlines certain plant sources of omega-3s, including their milligram amounts of ALA.

Note that ALA recommendations are 1.6 grams per day (1,600 milligrams) for men and 1.1 grams per day (1,100 milligrams) for women.[186] Per the World Health Organization (WHO), the general guidelines for EPA and DHA are a combined 200 to 500 milligrams.[189]

EPA and DHA are synthesized by microalgae. These fatty acids become incorporated into fish and krill that eat these microalgae, thus food sources of EPA and DHA include fish, fish oils, and krill oil.[186] Vegetarian sources of EPA and DHA can include microalgae oil.[172]

You'll also find EPA and DHA in fortified foods like eggs, milk, and yogurt.[188] See Chart 3.3 for common animal foods that you'll find sources of omega-3s, primarily with excellent sources of DHA and EPA.

3.2 - Plant Sources of Omega-3 Fatty Acids for a 3-Tablespoon Serving

Fat source	Calories (kcal)	Protein (g)	Carb (g)	Fats (g)	ALA (mg)	DHA (mg)	EPA (mg)
Hemp seeds	166	10	3	15	2605	0	0
Pumpkin seeds	158	7	3	2	29	0	0
Chia seeds	207	7	18	13	7582	0	0
Walnuts, chopped	145	3	3	14	2000	0	0
Sunflower seeds	153	5	6	14	5	0	1
Sesame seeds	155	5	6	13	102	0	0
Flaxseeds, ground	112	4	6	9	4791	0	0

Source: USDA Food Composition Database[62]

3.3 - Animal Sources of Omega-3 Fatty Acids for a 3-ounce Serving

Fat source	Cal (kcal)	Pro (g)	Carb (g)	Fats (g)	ALA (mg)	DHA (mg)	EPA (mg)
Salmon, farmed	175	19	0	11	0	1238	587
Salmon, wild	155	21	0	7	0	1215	349
Sardines	177	21	0	10	817	433	402
Shrimp	101	19	0	1	0	120	115
Light tuna, canned in water	73	17	0	1	2	167	24
Chicken breast	140	26	0	3	0	17	9
Conventional ground beef	149	17	0	9	31	0	0
Grass-fed ground beef	168	16	0	11	60	0	1

Source: USDA Food Composition Database[62]

NUTRITION TIP

Your brain and eyes will thank you if you eat more DHA because DHA adds to their structure to keep them healthy. Did you know that the brain is made up of nearly 60% fat, and that omega-3s aid your neurotransmitters? Include them regularly in your diet for a healthy mind and body!

Saturated Fat

As opposed to unsaturated fats, saturated fats are linked to increased levels of serum cholesterol and increased risk of cardiovascular disease and stroke.[30,31] It is recommended to limit intake of saturated fats to less than 7-10% of total calorie intake.[190] How does that look in your daily diet? For someone who needs 2,000 calories each day, 7-10% would equate to a 16-22 gram saturated fat limit.

Increasing plant-based foods and substituting them for animal foods automatically decreases many sources of saturated fats. Saturated fats are primarily found in high-fat animal products such as beef, chicken skin, whole milk, whole-milk cheese, and ice cream. Choosing leaner cuts of meat and lower-fat dairy decreases saturated fat intake. Saturated fat from food raises blood cholesterol more than cholesterol from food. Cholesterol is found only in animal foods.

3.4 - Common Amounts of Total Fat and Saturated Fat in Animal Foods				
Food	Serving amount	Total fat (g)	Total unsaturated fat (g)	Total saturated fat (g)
Beef	3 oz.	12	6	5
Chicken with skin	3 oz.	11	7	3
Whole milk	8 fl. oz.	8	2	5
Cheese	1 oz.	9	3	5
Ice cream	⅔ cup	10	3	7

Source: USDA Food Composition Database[62]

Rounded numbers are utilized resulting in averages. Other fractional additions aren't captured such as cholesterol and trans fats.

While the serving size of beef is 3 ounces, many restaurants typically serve 8 ounces or more (as a filet or even on a burger). An 8-ounce serving would contain a little over 13 grams of saturated fat. Add in 1 ounce of cheese on that burger, and you're already at 18 grams of saturated fat in just one meal. It adds up quickly, especially with the common portion sizes served while eating out.

Plant-based sources of saturated fat

Don't be fooled – saturated fats are present in some plant-based foods too! These include coconut products (which we'll go into more depth about a little later), palm oils, and various processed foods such as cakes, pastries, and packaged snacks.[190-192] There are two main types of oil made from the palm – palm oil and palm kernel oil. Palm oil is taken from the flesh of the palm fruit, while palm kernel oil is extracted from the seed/kernel within that fruit. Palm kernel oil has nearly 33% more saturated fat than palm oil – rivaling the saturated fat of coconut oil. The less refined versions of palm oil may provide a source of carotenoids and other beneficial plant compounds, though other oils lower in saturated fat are still the preferred oil option.[193,194] Keep these foods in mind to be conscious of the amounts of saturated fat you have each day, and consume them in moderation.

Trans Fats

The last main category of fats is trans fats. Trans fats can occur naturally, but they are primarily created through a chemical process that partially hydrogenates liquid vegetable oil to produce a fat that contains extra hydrogen atoms. This makes them solid at room temperature, giving the food enhanced shelf stability.

Up until 2015, trans fats were commonly found in vegetable shortening, margarine, baked goods, and various packaged and fried foods.[195] However, beginning in the early 1990s, research began to shed light on the many dangers of trans fats. Intake of trans fats is linked to increased LDL (bad) cholesterol and decreased HDL (good) cholesterol. Intake of trans fats is also linked to increased inflammation, insulin resistance, and risk of coronary heart disease.[195] In 2002, the Institute of Medicine recommended reducing intake of trans fats to as little as possible.[196] In 2006, the FDA required trans fat content to be disclosed on food labels. In 2015, the FDA revoked trans fat's "Generally Recognized As Safe" (GRAS) status, and ruled that by June 2019, trans fats could no longer be added to foods in the United States![195,196]

Other sources of trans fats

Aside from those that are chemically created, trans fats are also produced in the digestive tract of some animals, including sheep and cows. As a result, small amounts of trans fats are found in some meat and dairy products.[197] By following a plant-based eating pattern, you will further decrease the intake of these trans fats.

Recommended Ranges of Fat Intake

The International Olympic Committee's (IOC) recommended range for fat intake among athletes is 20-35% of total calorie intake and is the same value recommended for the general population.[19,176] Due to the important roles fat has in the human body, it is recommended that fat intake does not fall lower than 15-20% of total calories each day, with a maximum of 10% of that total intake from saturated fat.[78,176]

Omega-3 Fatty Acid Recommendations

Per the Academy of Nutrition and Dietetics, it is recommended that you consume 250-500 milligrams of EPA + DHA per day, and per the World Health Organization (WHO) it's 200-500 milligrams.[185] Use the omega-3 charts from earlier in this section to see how you can reach those levels. We'll give you a hint – eating fish like salmon, sardines, trout, or oysters two times per week will help you reach your target.

Calculating Your Fat Needs

If you want a target for your own daily fat needs, start with an estimation of the total calories you need or currently eat in a day. This is something you can find online for a very rough estimate. Keep in mind that an estimated *minimum* amount of calories you can use is 27-30 calories per kilogram of body weight.[79] Of course, meeting with an RDN will be best for individualized and professional guidance.

Based on our carbohydrate and protein guidelines previously provided in this guide, identify your carbohydrate and protein needs based on grams per kilogram of body weight. Then, allocate your remaining calorie needs to fat, making sure they don't fall below the 15-20% of total intake. If you are trying to make body composition changes or reach certain performance goals, this is another way an RDN can make sure you're maximizing your nutrition intake to meet those goals.

Should You Supplement with Omega-3s?

There is currently no consensus on the benefit of omega-3 supplementation for performance. However, some studies have found that it can reduce exercise-induced inflammation and oxidative stress post exercise.[198]

Omega-3 supplements may also play a role in improving airway function during exercise for those who suffer from exercise-induced bronchospasm.[58]

As vegans may have inadequate intake of omega-3s, supplementation for the vegan athlete may be even more beneficial.[172] Algal Oil Supplements can be used as a vegan source of omega-3s. A typical dose you may find is 600 milligrams of omega-3s – 360 milligrams of DHA and 180 milligrams of EPA.[199] Note that these levels may vary by manufacturer. You can also look for an omega-3 supplement that contains DHA derived from a micro-algae source in combination with ALA derived from seeds such as chia or flax.[198] Just make sure to be aware of dosing, as the FDA recommends that you don't exceed 3 grams per day of a combination of EPA and DHA, with 2 grams a day from supplements, unless instructed by your doctor, dietitian, or other trusted health care provider.[188]

Another interesting focus on omega-3 supplementation has targeted muscle protein synthesis. Researchers have seen that a dose of 2 grams per day of omega-3 supplementation may increase muscle protein synthesis. However, this response may be blunted if adequate protein is consumed after exercise, and a hypocaloric diet or immobilization delete these effects.[89,236,237] This muscle building response has also been seen in older adults.[238]

Coconut Oil: Facts vs. Fiction

Coconut oil is a plant-based fat that has recently been put in the spotlight in the health food world. When you break down the nutrient composition and explore what the research says, coconut oil may not deserve all the hype it gets on the internet and popular TV profiles.

Nutrient Profile

Coconut oil is 100% fat, but only contains trace levels of the heart healthy unsaturated fats.[200] In total, it is made up of 92% saturated fat.[201] The primary type of saturated fat present in coconut oil is lauric acid, which takes up about 45-53% of coconut oil.[202] Lauric acid is a 12-chain carbon fatty acid that in many studies has been linked to increased levels of LDL cholesterol.[200] LDL is the type of cholesterol that can lead to clogged arteries and increased cardiovascular disease risk.[203]

Medium Chain Triglycerides and Coconut Oil

 Medium chain triglycerides, or MCTs, are often brought into the coconut oil conversation. Structurally, MCTs are shorter than other fats and are 6-12 carbons in length. These MCTs include caprylic acid, capric acid, and lauric acid– though lauric acid can mimic the action of long-chain fatty acids instead and may not be as readily available. MCTs' unique structure allows them to follow a different digestive pathway than other fats, facilitating more rapid absorption and processing. While MCTs are naturally present in a few types of oils and fats including palm kernel oil, breast milk, whole cow's milk, goat's milk, and coconut oil, the level of the desirable MCTs in many of these oils and fats is low.[204]

Due to this alternative way our body processes MCTs, MCTs are believed to have health-promoting benefits for certain populations. MCT oil can be beneficial for individuals with certain gastrointestinal disorders and for those with fat malabsorption.[205] Research has also shown potential benefits of MCT oil in blood glucose management for people with type 2 diabetes and for improving cognition and memory among Alzheimer's patients.[205-207]

However, it is very important to note that the findings from these studies on MCT oil cannot be translated to the benefits of unrefined coconut oil, as the fatty acid composition is very different.[208] Unrefined coconut oil (virgin coconut oil) is the oil you will most often see on the shelves and is what is typically added to recipes claiming MCT benefits. This oil is the type with much lower amounts of the desirable MCTs, caprylic and capric acid.

Some coconut oils are refined to have higher amounts of caprylic and capric acids, and lower amounts of lauric acid. These oils are considered refined coconut oils and are liquid at room temperature rather than solid. For example, refined coconut oil may have 50% caprylic acid, 38% capric acid, and 7% lauric acid, compared to coconut oil that has about 15% of caprylic and capric acid combined, and 45-53% lauric acid.

Sometimes the refined coconut oil is processed even further, which is how MCT oil is made. This takes out even more of the lauric acid, and the caprylic and capric acids make up 92-100% of the oil, rather than about 85% as with the refined coconut oil.[209]

The range of values for MCT concentration among coconut oil, refined coconut oil, and MCTs is why it is not appropriate to extrapolate the benefits of pure MCT oil to coconut oil as a whole.[205] The key to remember is that all three are made up of primarily (if not all) saturated fat, which is why the American Heart Association (AHA) still recommends limiting intake of this fat source.[209] So don't go nuts with coconut oil! Use it as an occasional fat to increase flavor, but not as a go-to source for fuel.

MCT oil for the athlete

So how does this play into sports enhancement? While it is recommended to limit consumption of saturated fat, consuming 100% MCT oil may have benefits for athletes. Due to the different mechanism that the body uses to digest MCTs in comparison to other fatty acids, MCTs have been mentioned as another type of fuel for athletes. However, keep in mind that fuel intake is not necessary during exercise that is less than approximately 1.5 hours in duration since we have enough fuel reserves if we're fueling properly. This means that the majority of the population would not benefit from consuming MCTs during exercise. For endurance exercise, the situation is a bit different, because athletes need to consume fuel to exercise at their peak for extended periods of time. The research on the benefits of MCT during exercise are conflicting, but here are a few things to note:

- Many studies have found no benefits of MCT oil supplementation for the athlete, with some even finding negative effects.[211]
- MCTs can also cause gastrointestinal distress, so it is important to weigh the risks and benefits of their consumption.
- Some of them are expensive and are included within a supplement, which adds one more thing you have to evaluate. Combined with

cost, these are rarely utilized at the collegiate level. Some brands cost 20 times more than others for the same product! This means it can get quite pricey if you don't do your research.[209]

At this time, more research among human subjects is needed before determining the impact of MCT oil on the athlete.

The Ketogenic Diet

Whether or not to follow the Ketogenic Diet for your athletic performance is a no brainer. Remember the carbohydrate section, where you read carbohydrates are the primary source of energy for the brain? If you're an athlete who likes to think straight, avoid the ketogenic diet! The ketogenic diet is characterized by a diet rich in fat, moderate in protein, and very low in carbohydrate, with generally between 20-50 grams of carbohydrate intake per day. Non-starchy vegetables and small amounts of certain fruits are also generally included. It doesn't allow most fruit, vegetables, whole grains, or regular or sweet potatoes – which are foods we know are associated with longevity, packed with disease-fighting phytonutrients. Following the ketogenic diet causes the body to switch from using glucose as a primary source of fuel to using ketones as fuel. This use of ketones is a main factor of ketosis and is possible with the body's ability to generate energy from ketone bodies. These ketone bodies are produced in the liver from fat. The body will start to switch its fuel source after 3-4 days of glucose deprivation, however, achieving ketosis and staying in that metabolic state can take greater than a week.[212,213] Think of this as your body's survival mechanism when your brain and cell's preferred fuel sources aren't available.

For certain medical conditions like epilepsy, there are benefits of the ketogenic diet. In the early 1900s, 2-3 day periods of fasting were found to help reduce seizures.[214] The classic ketogenic diet was then discovered as a way to mimic similar responses in the body, while also making sure individuals were meeting calorie needs. Medication is now available, and most people with seizure disorders do not need a ketogenic diet. However, for those who are unresponsive to seizure medication, it can be a lifesaver. While the mechanism is still partly unknown, scientists believe it has something to do with the breakdown of carbohydrates and/or the impact of ketones on neurotransmitters.[214,21]

There have been some other studies examining the impact of this diet for people with type 2 diabetes and who are obese, and there have been

---

The Plant-Based Boost

107

positive associations with their improved blood lipid markers and weight loss. However, we can't take these studies that are done with very specific non-athlete populations and extend them to the generally healthy, active adult population. This is one of the key reasons why a lot of what we read online can be misleading! Remember, one finding with a specific population and a specific study protocol doesn't make it the gold standard for everyone, everywhere.

So what are the key takeaways? For healthy individuals who don't have specific medical reasons for following this diet, the emphasis on foods high in saturated fat contradicts the current recommendation by the AHA to limit intake of these foods. Additionally, the limited and restrictive nature of the keto diet may lead to feelings of deprivation and hunger, as well as increased risk of micronutrient deficiencies. For athletes, it's a definitive NO! As pointed out earlier, carbohydrate intake positively influences training sessions and athletic performance and low carbohydrate diets lower performance quality and recovery time. Studies that have trialed the ketogenic diet with athletes have found no performance benefit, and many studies have even seen negative effects on performance.[215] Longer-term studies are needed to fully understand the lasting impacts of the keto diet. Following diets like this may also increase the risk of disordered eating and it takes the fun out of something that should be enjoyed – food!

Part 4:
SPECIAL CONSIDERATIONS FOR VEGANS AND VEGETARIANS

Nutrients of Concern

D URING TRAINING, ATHLETES MAY HAVE an increased demand for specific nutrients. This increased demand can usually be met with food. Any nutrient deficiencies observed in athletes are likely to be the result of restricted food intake rather than increased requirements due to the effects of training.[216] A well-planned vegetarian or vegan diet can be superior for your long-term health while still optimizing your athletic performance. However, certain nutrients are limited in plant-based sources. It is important to pay attention to the following nutrients to ensure adequacy in your plant-focused diet: vitamin B12, calcium, vitamin D, iodine, iron, zinc, and omega-3s.[172] If you eat mostly plant-based foods, consider monitoring these nutrients for two weekdays and one weekend day to assess if you're meeting your needs. Looking for a good tracking form? Visit MelissasHealthyLiving.com. You can also work with a dietitian to evaluate your overall nutrient intake and help with balanced meal planning.

Although vegans or vegetarians aren't at unique risk for low iodine intake, it's included in this table, as sea salt has grown in popularity and is not typically fortified.

4.1 - Food Sources of Key Nutrients for Vegans and Vegetarians			
Nutrient	**RDA**	**Sources (per standard serving)**	**Amount from source**
Vitamin B12	2.4 mcg	1 Tbsp. nutritional yeast	5.9 mcg
		1 cup cheerios original	1.9 mcg
		1 cup low-fat plain yogurt	1.3 mcg
		4 oz. tempeh	0.16 mcg+
Calcium	1000 mg	3 oz. tofu	325 mg+
		1 cup 1% milk	305 mg
		3 Tbsp. chia seeds	228 mg
		1 cup raw kale	53 mg
		1 cup raw broccoli	43 mg

4.1 - Food Sources of Key Nutrients for Vegans and Vegetarians (Continued)			
Nutrient	RDA	Sources (per standard serving)	Amount from source
Vitamin D	600 IU	1 cup sliced Portobello mushrooms	976 IU
		1 cup fortified orange juice	137 IU
		1 cup fortified almond milk	101 IU
		1 large egg	41 IU
Iodine[217]	150 mcg	1 g or 1 sheet seaweed	16-2,984 mcg
		¼ tsp. iodized salt	71 mcg
		5 dried prunes	13 mcg
Iron	8 mg (men) 18 mg (women)	½ cup uncooked oats	1.8 mg
		1 cup cheerios original	8.1 mg
		½ cup tofu	3.3 mg
		1 cup cooked spinach	6.4 mg
		1 cup cooked kidney beans	5.2 mg
		½ cup cooked lentils	3.3 mg
		¼ cup pumpkin seeds	2.4 mg
Zinc	11 mg (men) 8 mg (women)	1 cup cheerios original	3.8 mg
		¼ cup pumpkin seeds	2.5 mg
		1 cup low-fat plain yogurt	2.2 mg
		¼ cup dry, roasted cashews	1.9 mg
		1 cup cooked green peas	1.9 mg
		½ cup cooked chickpeas	1.3 mg
Omega-3s* (ALA)	1.6 g (men) 1.1 g (women)	3 Tbsp. chia seeds	7.6 g
		3 Tbsp. ground flaxseeds	4.8 g
		3 Tbsp. walnuts, chopped	2.0 g

Sources: USDA Food Composition Database and Office of Dietary Supplements[65,94]

*AI (adequate intake) for omega-3

+varies by brand and fermentation methods

Vitamin B12

What it does & why it's needed:

Vitamin B12 is necessary for red blood cell production and nerve, heart, and muscle function. It is also involved in metabolism and the production of your DNA and serotonin.[79] Serotonin is a biochemical messenger that coordinates activities in the central nervous system, which affects mood and behavior.[218]

How much you need:
Adults, both male, and female, need 2.4 micrograms daily.

Food sources:
B12 is rarely found in plants. Even lacto-ovo-vegetarians (those who include milk and eggs) may be at risk for deficiency due to vitamin losses during pasteurization, cooking, and processing of dairy products. Vegan athletes should have their blood B12 levels monitored annually. Supplementation is often necessary. You can also try nutritional yeast for a B12 boost – in just ¼ cup you get 240% of your daily needs. It is a great item to add to your pantry (even if you're an omnivore!). It's also an excellent source of many other B vitamins and packs a punch with 8 grams of protein per ¼ cup. It's a vegan food, with a cheesy taste, making it great to add to pretty much anything. It's also yummy in popcorn or in homemade cashew cheese.

Deficiency:
Deficiency can cause motor dysfunction, slowed reaction times, and anemia. Prolonged deficiency may cause irreversible neurological damage.[172]

Toxicity:
Toxicity is rarely an issue as B12 is a water-soluble vitamin; therefore, excess is excreted in the urine.[219]

Unique characteristics:
Insufficient B12 may mask a folic acid deficiency due to B12's role in converting folate to a useable form in the body. In this case, blood levels of folate may appear high, but it will only be due to the lack of B12 halting folate's conversion.[220]

Calcium

What it does & why it's needed:
Calcium is vital for bone health and muscle contractions.

How much you need:
The RDA for calcium is 1,000 milligrams. Although athletes may have

increased calcium loss via perspiration, 1,000 milligrams should still be plenty to satisfy their requirements.[172]

Food sources:
While dairy products may be the richest sources of calcium, plant sources such as dark, leafy greens and tofu can provide adequate calcium in lieu of dairy.

Deficiency:
Low dietary calcium is associated with greater fracture risk. Most people reach peak bone mass around age 30, so it is crucial to ensure optimal intake to have good bone reserves as you age.

Toxicity:
Too much calcium, especially from high doses of supplements can cause calcium to deposit outside your bones and into other areas of your body – most commonly in arteries. This poses a threat to cardiovascular health; therefore, calcium supplementation should be consumed in small doses and only if your healthcare provider deems it necessary.

Unique characteristics:
It is hypothesized that vegans' bodies may adapt to have higher calcium absorption rates than non-vegans to compensate for lower intakes. Sufficient intake of vitamin D is also known to boost calcium absorption.[172]

Vitamin D

What it does & why it's needed:
It is well established that vitamin D plays a critical role in bone health and immune function, which can keep athletes healthy and avoid missing practice due to illness. Additionally, the Academy of Nutrition and Dietetics cites emerging evidence relating vitamin D intake to injury prevention, muscle growth, and inflammation reduction.[78]

How much you need:
The RDA for vitamin D is 600 International Units. The safe upper limit for adults is 4,000 International Units, though if treated for low blood levels, the repletion dosage will exceed this.

Food sources:
With adequate sunlight exposure, vitamin D will be synthesized by our skin. Supplementation may be necessary due to the geographic location if it is not compensated for in the diet.[172] There are a few food sources that

contain vitamin D, including but not limited to UV-treated mushrooms, fortified orange juice, and egg yolks.

Deficiency:
The best way to check your vitamin D levels for a possible deficiency is through a blood test to measure plasma vitamin D. If your levels are found to be inadequate, your healthcare provider can help you determine proper dosing for supplementation.

Toxicity:
While no toxicity incidents have been reported from endogenous vitamin D, excess supplemental vitamin D can cause hypercalcemia and may lead to calcified tissues and vessels due to its role in calcium absorption.[20]

Unique characteristic:
Some studies suggest that a vitamin D deficiency in athletes may impair muscle strength and oxygen consumption, perhaps due in part to its role in calcium metabolism.

Iodine

What it does & why it's needed:
Iodine is a trace element that naturally occurs in some foods, can be used to fortify foods and is also used in most multivitamin and mineral supplements. It's an essential component of thyroid hormones and is involved in protein synthesis, metabolic activity, and other enzymatic reactions.[172]

How much you need:
For males and females 19 years old or older, the RDA is 150 micrograms. Women who are pregnant or lactating have a higher RDA, 220 micrograms and 290 micrograms, respectively.[217]

Food sources:
Seaweed provides one of the highest sources, though varieties of seaweed may have different iodine amounts.[217,221] Many sources of iodine are animal-based, including fish, dairy, and eggs, so it is important for vegan athletes to seek other sources. Plant-based sources include, but are not limited to, cranberries, potatoes, prunes, navy beans, fortified grains, and iodized salt.[172,217] Iodized salt is one of the easiest ways to make sure you are consuming adequate iodine as you can add it to dishes and sprinkle it on food – especially to replenish electrolytes lost after exercise. The content of iodine in food can also vary based on the iodine content of the soil in which it was grown.[80,172]

Deficiency:

Insufficient iodine can lead to a decreased production of thyroid hormone concentrations.[217] Low levels of iodine typically present as goiter – a swelling of the thyroid gland, which presents as an enlarged neck. Another common symptom is decreased mental capacity.[217]

Intake and quantity of goitrogens is another factor that can lead to deficiency if iodine intake is inadequate.[222] Foods that contain goitrogens include cruciferous vegetables like broccoli and cauliflower, as well as soy, cabbage, and others.[217] However, this shouldn't be a concern if your iodine levels and intake are adequate.[80]

NUTRITION TIP

Looking for ways to boost your iodine without a supplement?
- Make some veggie sushi wrapped in seaweed.
- Sprinkle iodized salt on your roasted veggies.
- Enjoy a cup of low-fat yogurt.

Some vegans may need to consider supplementation to reach adequate iodine intake. If you're concerned that you aren't getting enough iodine in your daily diet, meet with an RDN for a proper analysis and action plan. Iodine supplements can interfere with specific medications, so make sure to mention any prescription medications during your appointment.

Toxicity:

The Tolerable Upper Intake Levels for iodine for men and women 19 years of age or older is 1,100 micrograms. Around ¼ teaspoon of salt has 68 micrograms.[62] Too much iodine can lead to elevated Thyroid Stimulating Hormone (TSH) levels, hypothyroidism, and goiter.[217] Ironically, these are very similar symptoms you'll see with iodine deficiency, which is why it's important to understand and be aware of how much iodine is in the foods you eat.

Unique characteristics:

Many salts like sea salt and pink Himalayan sea salt have become more popular in the past several years, partly due to their added benefits of essential minerals and taste. However, these salts, in addition to Kosher salts, typically aren't fortified with iodine and may take away a valuable and simple source of iodine for a vegan's daily needs.

Iron

What it does & why it's needed:

Iron is an essential component of metabolism and heart health. It's one of the parts of hemoglobin, the substance in red blood cells that carries oxygen. Making sure you consume enough iron will help ensure optimal oxygen delivery to the muscles.[223] Sufficient iron is also needed to prevent anemia, which can hinder an athlete's muscle work capacity and cause them to feel winded sooner since the blood is less oxygenated.[224] Distance runners show an increase in hemoglobin in the blood, and increased myoglobin and cytochromes in the muscle cells. Why does this matter for iron status? All three compounds need iron in order to be formed! To achieve the adaptations you are aiming for, you want to reach your daily iron needs.

How much you need:

Men need about 8 milligrams daily, women ages 19-50 need 18 milligrams, and women over 50 years of age need 9 milligrams.[223] Athletes need more iron due to heavy sweating, increased demand for growth in the number of red blood cells and small blood vessels, increased blood loss in urine and the gastrointestinal tract, with extreme events resulting in higher losses.[225] Damage from injury and "foot strike" (damage to red blood cells in feet from hard surfaces) also increases iron loss. Sometimes athletes need 1.3 to 1.7 times higher dietary iron intake due to increased iron losses during a vigorous sweat session, higher rates of red blood cell destruction, and exercise-induced inflammation.[226,227] To accurately evaluate your needs, get your iron levels checked by your healthcare provider. Women of reproductive age should monitor their intake and have iron status checked annually. Supplementation may be indicated.[224]

Food sources:

There are two main types of iron – heme and non-heme:

- non-heme iron is in plant and animal sources as well as fortified foods
- heme iron is only found in animal products and is more readily absorbed than non-heme

The lower absorption rate of non-heme iron can be compensated by increased intake of iron- and zinc-rich foods such as pumpkin seeds and legumes, soaking beans prior to cooking, pairing a vitamin C source with your plant meals higher in iron, and avoiding calcium supplements or calcium-rich foods within a 2-hour window of eating.[172] High vitamin C foods include oranges, kiwi, guava, strawberries, papaya, red, green and yellow peppers, broccoli, kohlrabi, snow peas, grapefruit and mango.[62,228]

4.2 - Plant and Animal Sources of Iron			
Plant sources	Iron (mg)	Animal sources	Iron (mg)
Fortified breakfast cereals, 1 cup	up to 18	Wild oyster, 3 oz.	7.8
Spinach, 1 cup, cooked	6.4	Sardines, 3 oz.	4.4
Lentils, ½ cup, cooked	3.3	Ground beef, 3 oz.	2.1
Tofu, ½ cup, cooked	3.3	Tuna, 3 oz. canned in water	0.97
Pumpkin seeds, ¼ cup	2.4	Egg, 1 whole	0.96
White beans, ½ cup, canned	1.8	Chicken breast, 3 oz.	0.8

Source: USDA Food Composition Database[65]

Deficiency:

Signs of deficiency include fatigue, dizziness, pale skin, feeling cold, headaches, and shortness of breath. The best test of iron status is serum ferritin. If you get bloodwork done, make sure serum ferritin is checked; don't rely on a complete blood count known as a CBC.[229] The International Olympic Committee (IOC) Consensus Statement on Periodic Health Evaluation of Elite Athletes recommends that females have their iron status checked during periodic health evaluations.

Toxicity:

The safest way to ensure you are meeting your iron needs is to consume iron-rich foods alongside vitamin C-rich foods to maximize absorption. Iron supplements can have dangerous effects when consumed in excess. Many athletes take supplemental iron incorrectly or for too long which can lead to toxicity. Take appropriate doses (based on lab results), recheck levels after 8-12 weeks, and then drop to a maintenance dose if your levels have been corrected. An excess of iron can be a pro-oxidant and could potentially increase heart disease risk, gastric upset, or be harmful if an individual has undiagnosed hemochromatosis.[230]

Unique characteristics:

For women who need to boost iron intake, you can cook with an iron skillet. While you can use the skillet with the whole family, be aware of the fact that most males only need 8 milligrams of iron a day. Simply cooking pasta sauce in the skillet can increase the iron content by more than 5 milligrams, partly because the vitamin C from the sauce helps absorption of iron![231] This is something to keep in mind, though it isn't of too big of a concern since the upper limit for iron is 45 milligrams per day. It is difficult to achieve these levels without large amounts of red meat or supplementation. For now, even more reason to grab iron-rich plant sources!

HEALTH INSIGHT

Low energy availability, also known as relative energy deficiency in sports (RED-S), occurs when you are not consuming the amount of calories your body needs to meet the demands of your exercise. This can occur through inadequate intake, or excessive exercise.[232] It can occur in both males and females and is usually accompanied by other health issues such as lack of menstrual cycles in females, weakened immune system, bone health, and others.[232] For those on oral contraceptives, it may be masked. This is why it's key to work with an RDN, especially for more elite athletes.

This is a popular topic in sports nutrition and can happen due to reduced hunger from intense training, difficulty eating enough to meet energy needs, or trying to meet certain body composition goals for competition.

As a general rule of thumb, here are some simple calculations you can make to see if you're reaching your needs, based on a 50-80 kilogram (110-176-pound) individual:[79]

- Exercise 30-40 minutes, 3x/week: 25-35 kcals/kg/day
- Exercise 2-3 hours, 5-6x/week OR 3-6 hours (in 1-2 workouts), 5-6x/week: 40-70 kcals/kg/day

The ranges are quite large, which is why meeting with an RDN can be the missing link for your performance success.

Zinc

What it does & why it's needed:
Zinc plays an integral role in immune health. It can impact cell replication through DNA and protein synthesis.[20] Additionally, zinc can also impact cardiovascular and muscle endurance.[233]

How much you need:
Men require 11 milligrams daily, while women only need 8 milligrams.[234]

Food sources:
Zinc is found in both plant and animal sources, but as with iron, animal sources may be more bioavailable. Protein appears to enhance its bioavailability while supplemental folic acid, iron, calcium, copper, and magnesium may inhibit absorption. It is important to note that this was only found in supplements, not from food sources of the aforementioned nutrients.[172]

Breakfast cereal, baked beans, fruit, yogurt, and cashews are good plant-based sources of zinc. High animal sources include oysters, beef, and crab.[234]

Deficiency:
If you find that normal cuts and scrapes are taking longer than usual to heal, feel continually under the weather, or lost your sense of taste, you may be zinc deficient.

Toxicity:
Zinc in excess can cause headaches, abdominal cramps, and nausea. Prolonged intake beyond one's needs can result in a copper deficiency and neurological damage. Using a zinc nasal spray can impact your sense of smell if used inappropriately.[20]

Omega-3s

What they do & why they're needed:
Omega-3 fatty acids are the anti-inflammatory counterparts to omega-6 fatty acids. Omega-3s are crucial for brain and eye development during pregnancy. They continue to be important for brain health and an integral component of your body cells.[188]

How much you need:
The adequate intake of ALA omega-3s is set at 1.6 grams for men and 1.1

grams for women. Although as previously noted there is not a consensus on omega-3 recommendations in athletes. It's recommended not to exceed 2 grams of omega-3s in supplemental form per day.[186] The World health Organization (WHO) recommends about 1-2 servings of fatty fish per week, such as salmon or mackerel. A 3-ounce serving of wild or farmed salmon has around 2,000 milligrams. So if you were to eat fatty fish 1-2 times per week, you would meet the WHO recommendation of 200-500 milligrams of omega-3s per day through food.[235,236]

Food sources:
Salmon gained super food popularity due to its incredibly high omega-3 content. However, microalgae oil, chia, flax, hemp, and walnuts are all nutrient-dense foods containing high levels of omega-3s.

Deficiency:
Signs of omega-3 deficiency include dry and irritated skin.[186]

Toxicity:
Consuming excess omega-3 supplements may cause fishy breath or digestive issues. It can also interact with blood clotting medications. As always, it is best to consume nutrients via the diet. Keep in mind that overdoing supplementation with omega-3s can suppress the immune system, which is why it's wise to follow the recommendations of no more than 2 grams per day of EPA/DHA supplementation.[199] If you're considering a supplement, work with a dietitian for a safe brand and amount.

Unique characteristic:
Due to their ability to reduce cellular inflammation, new research is exploring how omega-3s may attenuate muscle soreness and decrease post-exercise muscle damage from resistance (eccentric) exercise, though more research is needed.[89]

After accounting for the nutrients discussed above, athletes and avid exercisers that are vegans or vegetarians can achieve comparable performance to their omnivorous counterparts. Plant-based diets offer unique benefits to athletes because of their dietary antioxidants, phytochemicals, fiber, and vitamins and minerals. It is theorized that the anti-inflammatory nature of plant-based diets can help in recovery and longevity.[13,239] Keep an eye out for more research involving plant-based diets and fitness.

FOOD FEATURE: LENTILS

Lentils are an affordable, versatile option to add to your meal prep repertoire. Make a big batch at the start of the week and add them to salads, soups, stir-fry dishes, tacos, and more!

LENTIL FACTS (per ½ cup, cooked):

- Excellent source of iron[62]
- Excellent source of folate[62]
- Good source of potassium[62]
- About ⅓ of DV for fiber[62]
- Good source of thiamin[62]
- Come in a variety of colors that offer different phytonutrients
- Work well as a ground meat substitute in Bolognese sauce or in place of ground beef in sloppy Joes. Check out the companion recipe book for tasty ways to eat lentils!

Lentils can help lower cholesterol, improve nitrogen balance, and lower blood glucose levels. They also contain resistant starch which feeds healthful bacteria protecting colon cells.[27]

Nutrition Values Source: USDA Food Composition Database[62]

A Healthy Balance of the Macronutrients

Now that you're more familiar with the three macronutrients – carbohydrates, protein, and fat – and the recommended amounts for each, you may be wondering if there is a certain eating pattern that you can follow to make sure you hit all of your targets. While we don't typically promote diets, there are a few out there that have more of a focus on quality foods rather than the quickest weight loss fix. Just keep in mind, the type of diet you eat shouldn't take up a huge amount of mental energy. It should be part of a healthy lifestyle that brings you joy as an athlete and individual. Once you adapt to new changes and adopt diet principles that work for you, as well as a snack and meal list that you can recycle (full of tasty meals you like and filled with key nutrients you need), eating healthy becomes easy and isn't a chore.

Have you heard of the DASH Diet (Dietary Approaches to Stop Hypertension), the Mediterranean Diet, the MIND Diet, and/or the Nordic Diet? They are all pretty similar to each other with a few small differences in their core "health" beliefs. If you're eating a pattern similar to any of these, you'll be eating a variety of colorful foods and healthy fats. Here are the key facts for you to know.

The Mediterranean Diet

This isn't so much a diet as it is an eating style, and moderation is key here. Who wouldn't want to eat like the Greeks and other Mediterranean natives? This plant food focus with lean animal protein makes it easier to find balance. It includes:

- fruits and vegetables
- grains (including breads), nuts, seeds, and legumes
- proteins – fish and poultry are key – red meat and eggs also find their way in
- dairy – yogurt, and cheese take the spotlight here
- healthy oils – can you say olive oil?

The diverse colors and variety of mostly plant-based foods give you a range of phytonutrients that can help protect your DNA and fight off diseases. These foods are typically not very processed, thus they're naturally low in sodium. As with anything else – start small. If you know you can improve on one of these areas, make it your highlight and continue focusing on it until you feel confident it's become more of a habit than a chore.

The DASH Diet

As mentioned before, DASH stands for **D**ietary **A**pproaches to **S**top **H**ypertension. While that may sound a bit medical, this food approach has been used for much more than a technique to stop hypertension. Just like the Mediterranean Diet, the DASH diet is more of a lifestyle modification than anything else. One of the keys is to reduce excess sodium in the diet to adhere to the Dietary Guidelines for Americans of <2,300 milligrams per day for the average American (or <1,500 milligrams if on a very low sodium DASH diet*).[240] As with the Mediterranean Diet, the focus is still on lots of fruits and veggies, lean poultry, grains, nuts, seeds, legumes, and healthy fats/oils. The only big difference we see is that they don't quite LOVE olive oil as much as the Mediterranean Diet.[241]

*If you are an endurance athlete or are a salty sweater, don't let their push for low sodium scare you away! You can replace the electrolytes you lost in your sweat, including sodium, during exercise by adding in some table salt (with iodine). Head back to the hydration section if you want some number comparisons.

The MIND Diet

This stands for **M**editerranean-DASH Diet **I**ntervention for **N**euro-degenerative **D**elay. As you can gather from the name, this is very similar to the Mediterranean and DASH diet (these two are alike, to begin with!), but it has a few more modifications that are specific to findings in the dementia field of research. The basis of the diet is to push plant-based foods and limit the intake of animal foods and foods that are high in saturated fat.[242] You'll also notice that dairy isn't included on the list of healthy foods (as it is with the DASH diet). If you're going to include poultry, but not dairy, you could be missing out on some beneficial probiotics and a quick and convenient way to get protein and leucine. If you want to include dairy, the diets above may be a better fit. The MIND diet has a scoring pattern based on the classification of healthy and unhealthy food groups as they relate to the research findings on the effects on brain health. They are as follows:

Healthy: green leafy vegetables, other vegetables, nuts, berries, whole grains, seafood, poultry, olive oil, wine

Unhealthy: red meats, butter, stick margarine, cheese, pastries and sweets, fried/fast food

The Nordic Diet

This diet is most comparable to the Mediterranean diet with an emphasis on hearty whole grains, especially barley, oats, and rye. The diet is also abundant in berries. Once again, there is a large focus on plant-based foods. The Greeks may disapprove since olive oil is replaced with canola oil (or rapeseed oil). One of the best parts of this diet that isn't emphasized with others is the focus on local foods and supporting local vendors.[243] It really gets to the heart of why plant-based eating is so fantastic. Not only are you benefiting your body, but you're also benefiting the world around you that offers the opportunity to exercise outdoors and enjoy all that nature has to offer!

Alcohol

Regular alcohol intake can lead to fatigue, nutrition and sleep compromise, and poor athletic performance. Choosing a diet plan with no, or occasional, alcohol content will likely have a positive impact on performance.

Keep in mind that whichever diet you choose, new research shows that ethanol, the alcohol found in drinks, is a recognized carcinogen that may lead to DNA damage. Per the American Institute for Cancer Research (AICR), alcohol may also reduce folate absorption or help potential carcinogens enter the cell. Regular consumption of alcohol increases the risk of several cancers including the mouth, pharynx, larynx, esophagus, liver, breast, stomach, and colorectum.[244] If you do drink, try cutting back the number of days per week, and don't exceed 2 standard drinks for men and 1 for women per day. This includes 12 fluid ounces of regular beer (5% alcohol), 8-9 ounces of malt liquor (6-9% alcohol), 5 ounces of table wine (12% alcohol) or 1.5 fluid ounces of 80-proof distilled spirits such as whiskey, gin, rum, vodka, or tequila (40% alcohol).[244,245]

A Plant-Based Diet for Athletes – What's on Your Plate?

The International Olympic Committee (IOC) Athlete's Plate is an excellent guide to eating for easy, moderate and hard training/race days.[246] Adjusting the composition of your meal plans based off of your exercise level is key to optimal fueling.

Eating Guidelines per the IOC[246]
- **Easy:** "An easy day may contain just an easy workout or tapering without the need to load up for competition with energy and nutrients. Easy day meals may also apply to athletes trying to lose weight and athletes in sports requiring less energy (calories) due to the nature of their sport."
- **Moderate:** "A moderate day could be one where you train twice but focus on technical skill in one workout and on endurance in the other. The moderate day should be your baseline from where you adjust your plate down (easy) or up (hard/race)."
- **Hard:** "A hard day contains at least two workouts that are relatively hard or is a competition day. If your competition requires extra fuel from carbohydrates, use this plate to load up in the days before, throughout, and after the event day."

THE PLANT-BASED BOOST

ATHLETE'S PLATE:
EASY TRAINING / WEIGHT MANAGMENT

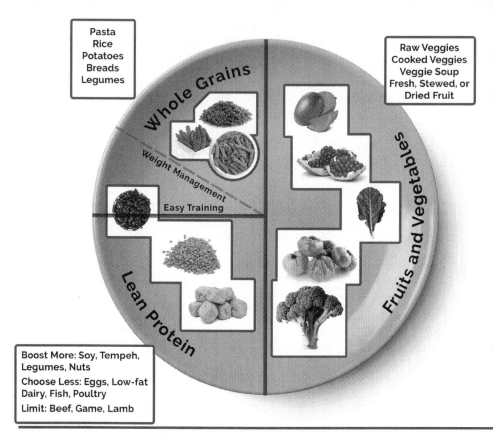

Pasta
Rice
Potatoes
Breads
Legumes

Raw Veggies
Cooked Veggies
Veggie Soup
Fresh, Stewed, or
Dried Fruit

Whole Grains

Weight Management

Easy Training

Fruits and Vegetables

Lean Protein

Boost More: Soy, Tempeh,
Legumes, Nuts

Choose Less: Eggs, Low-fat
Dairy, Fish, Poultry

Limit: Beef, Game, Lamb

Beverage	Flavors	Fats	Omega-3 Boost
Water	Herbs/Spices	Avocado	Walnuts
Dairy/Nondairy Beverage (vitamin D and calcium fortified)	Salt/Pepper	1 Tsp. of Healthy Oil	Chia Seeds
	Lemon/Lime Juice	Nuts	Tuna
	Vinegar	Seeds	Salmon
Diluted Juice	Salsa	Healthy Butter Substitute	Sardines
Coffee	Mustard	Cheese and Butter in Moderation	
Tea	Ketchup		

Adapted from The Athlete's Plates. The Athlete's Plate is a collaboration between the United States Olympic Committee Sport Dietitians and the University of Colorado (UCCS) Sport Nutrition Graduate Program.

Melissa Halas MA, RDN, CDE

THE PLANT-BASED BOOST

ATHLETE'S PLATE: MODERATE TRAINING DAY

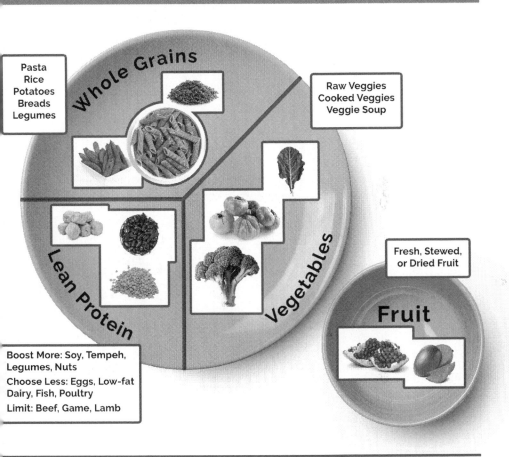

Pasta
Rice
Potatoes
Breads
Legumes

Whole Grains

Raw Veggies
Cooked Veggies
Veggie Soup

Lean Protein

Vegetables

Fresh, Stewed,
or Dried Fruit

Fruit

Boost More: Soy, Tempeh,
Legumes, Nuts

Choose Less: Eggs, Low-fat
Dairy, Fish, Poultry

Limit: Beef, Game, Lamb

Beverage	Flavors	Fats	Omega-3 Boost
Water	Herbs/Spices	Avocado	Walnuts
Dairy/Nondairy Beverage (vitamin D and calcium fortified)	Salt/Pepper	1 Tbsp. of Healthy Oil	Chia Seeds
	Lemon/Lime Juice	Nuts	Tuna
	Vinegar	Seeds	Salmon
Diluted Juice	Salsa	Healthy Butter Substitute	Sardines
Coffee	Mustard	Cheese and Butter in Moderation	
Tea	Ketchup		

Adapted from The Athlete's Plates. The Athlete's Plate is a collaboration between the United States Olympic Committee Sport Dietitians and the University of Colorado (UCCS) Sport Nutrition Graduate Program.

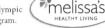

THE **PLANT-BASED BOOST**

ATHLETE'S PLATE: HARD TRAINING/RACE DAY

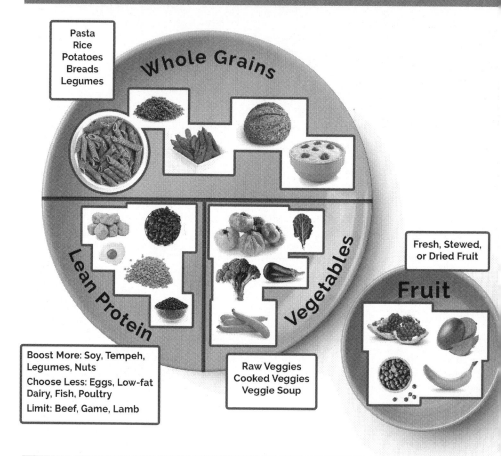

Pasta
Rice
Potatoes
Breads
Legumes

Whole Grains

Lean Protein

Vegetables

Fruit

Fresh, Stewed,
or Dried Fruit

Boost More: Soy, Tempeh,
Legumes, Nuts
Choose Less: Eggs, Low-fat
Dairy, Fish, Poultry
Limit: Beef, Game, Lamb

Raw Veggies
Cooked Veggies
Veggie Soup

Beverage	Flavors	Fats	Omega-3 Boost
Water	Herbs/Spices	Avocado	Walnuts
Dairy/Nondairy Beverage (vitamin D and calcium fortified)	Salt/Pepper	2 Tbsp. of Healthy Oil	Chia Seeds
	Lemon/Lime Juice	Nuts	Tuna
	Vinegar	Seeds	Salmon
Diluted Juice	Salsa	Healthy Butter Substitute	Sardines
Coffee	Mustard	Cheese and Butter in Moderation	
Tea	Ketchup		

Adapted from The Athlete's Plates. The Athlete's Plate is a collaboration between the United States Olympic Committee Sport Dietitians and the University of Colorado (UCCS) Sport Nutrition Graduate Program.

melissa's
HEALTHY LIVING

Melissa Halas MA, RDN, CDE

Part 5:
PHYTONUTRIENTS

Phytonutrients and Healthy Components of Plant-Based Proteins

Y OU MAY HAVE HEARD THE term phytochemicals, also known as phytonutrients. Remember this by the term fight-o-chemical because they fight off disease. They have recently gained a lot more popularity in the media – and rightfully so! Phytochemicals are biologically active compounds of plant origin that provide functional benefits beyond basic nutrition.[247] Sounds complicated, right? But it's simple! They have powerful antioxidant activity that helps the body fight against cancer, enhance the immune system, protect against environmental toxins, decrease inflammation, and soreness, and help promote healthy bacteria in the digestive tract.[151]

While fruits and vegetables are well known for being rich in phytochemicals, it's less widely known that whole grains and legumes are also great sources of these beneficial compounds. Including a combination of fruits, vegetables, whole grains, beans, herbs, and spices in the diet provides more than just energy – it also helps enhance health and immunity. So, when you eat the whole rainbow, don't forget to include white (onion), brown (cinnamon), and black foods (blackberries). Although most animal-based proteins have higher biological value to fulfill athletes' protein needs, plant-based proteins have phytochemical value. Be sure to include plant-based proteins in the form of colorful produce in everyday meals to help you perform better as an athlete and contribute to your general wellbeing and disease prevention.

Phytochemicals – The Basics

Are you getting in at least four to five different colors from plant-based foods each day? They all have important phytochemicals. Each color provides a different body benefit. Tens of thousands of different phytochemicals exist, and they are part of the plant's natural defense mechanisms. When we consume them, their antibacterial and antiviral properties also help to defend our bodies. Many phytochemicals can act as antioxidants, potentially decreasing our risk of developing cancer, atherosclerosis, and type 2 diabetes. Some may also decrease our LDL cholesterol, inhibit tumor growth, and aid with preventing osteoporosis.[20]

When we said there are hundreds of phytochemicals, we weren't kidding.

Here is a cheat-sheet chart **(5.1 - Phytochemicals Classification on page 129)** of some of the main ones that you can keep handy if you ever hear some phytochemical names and want to see how they fit into the bigger picture.[109]

SNACK ON THIS!

Pop-pop-pop! Popcorn! Popcorn is a whole grain packed with polyphenols. Toss with olive oil, parmesan cheese or nutritional yeast and Italian seasonings for a tasty snack![249]

Phytochemicals can have other surprising benefits. Here are just a few examples:

1. Polyphenols, like the flavonoid catechin found in tea, may promote anti-inflammatory responses.[248] Chronic inflammation contributes to the leading causes of death. Some polyphenols also lower risks of cancer and may protect you from gum disease too!
2. Bioflavonoids found in citrus may help prevent erectile dysfunction.
3. Carotenoids, the pigments found in orange fruits and vegetables, have been associated with an increased immune function in the body.
4. Glucosinolates, found in cruciferous vegetables (cabbage and Brussels sprouts), have tumor-fighting properties.
5. Anthocyanins found in blueberries, cherries, red cabbage, and radishes can boost cognitive function and decrease muscle soreness (tart cherries and watermelon come into play here – more on this later).[109]

In addition, many phytochemicals can help improve interneuron signaling (neuron to neuron communication) and increase neurogenesis (a process which by new neurons are formed in the brain) helping to decrease neurodegenerative disease. To help keep your mind sharp, this is another reason to boost plant-based fight-o-chemicals!

Check out our chart **(5.2 - Phytochemical Benefits on page 130-132)** to learn about all the possible benefits and plant sources of popular (or widely-studied) phytochemicals.[250–252]

Polyphenols	Carotenoids	Glucosinolates	Polysaccharides	Lectins	Terpenes
• Flavanones	• Beta-carotene	• Glucoiberin	• Cellulose	• Concanavalin A	• Cinerin I
• Flavones	• Cryptoxanthin	• Progoitrin	• Hemicellulose	• Wheat germ agglutinin	• Geraniol
• Dihydroflavonols	• Lutein	• Sinigrin	• Arabinoxylans	• Ricin	• Calotropin
• Flavonols	• Zeaxanthin	• Gluconapoleiferin	• Arabinogalactans	• Peanut agglutinin	• Strigol
• Flavan-3-ols		• Glucoraphanin	• Polyfructose	• Soybean agglutinin	• Caulerpenyne
• Anthocyanidins	**Alkaloids**	• Glucoalyssin	• Polydextrose		• Farnesane
• Isoflavones	• Ajmaline	• Glucocapparin	• Methyl cellulose	**Capsaicinoids**	• Squalene
• Proanthocyanidins	• Berberine	• Glucobrassicin	• Inulin	• Capsaicin	
• Phenols	• Caffeine	• Neoglucobrassicin	• Oligofructans	• Dihydrocapsaicin	**Betalains**
• Benzoic acids	• Camptothecin	• Glucosinalbin	• Oligosaccharide	• Homocapsaicin	• Betalain
• Hydrolyzable tannins	• Cocaine	• Glucotropaeolin	• Gums	• Nonivamide	• Betaxanthins
• Acetophenones	• Codeine	• Gluconasturtiin	• Mucilages		• Vulgaxanthin
• Phenylacetic acids	• Hyoscyamine		• Pectins		• Miraxanthin
• Cinnamic acids	• Irinotecan	**Polyacetylenes**			• Portulaxanthin
• Coumarins	• Morphine	• Falcarinol	**Allium compounds**		• Indicaxanthin
• Benzophenones	• Nicotine	• Falcarindiol	• Methiin		
• Xanthones	• Noscapine	• Panaxydiol	• Propiin	**Chlorophyll**	
• Stilbenes	• Oxycodone	• Oenanthetol	• Isoalliin		
• Chalcones	• Oxymorphone				
• Lignans	• Papaverine				
• Secoiridoids					

Adapted from Figure 2.1 Classification of phytochemicals

5.2 - Phytochemical Benefits

Phytochemical(s)	Plant source	Possible benefits/protection
Carotenoids (Beta-carotene, Lycopene, Lutein, Zeaxanthin)	Apricots, broccoli, cantaloupe, carrot, leafy greens, oranges, sweet potatoes, tomatoes, watermelon, winter squash	Anti-bacterial Antioxidant Inhibits cancer cell growth Strengthens immune function
• Beta-carotene	Cantaloupe melons, citrus fruit, collard, lettuce, mangos, orange carrot, peppers, pumpkin, purple carrot, spinach, sweet potato, turnip	Anti-cancer Mitigates free radical damage in the human eye Protects against CVD
• Lycopene	Eggplant, papaya, pink grapefruit, red carrot, red guava, red pepper, tomatoes, watermelon	Cancer (lowers risk of prostate cancer) Diabetes Protects against CVD
• Lutein, Zeaxanthin	Avocado, broccoli, Brussels sprouts, collard greens, corn, leafy greens, amaranth, kale, peas, purple carrot, spinach, squash, zucchini, eggs*	Cancer (colon cancer) Cataracts Diabetes Macular degeneration (absorbs blue and UV light)
Organosulfur Compounds (Indoles, Glucosinolates, Isothiocyanates, Sulforaphane)	Chives, cruciferous vegetables (broccoli, Brussels sprouts, cabbage, cauliflower, collard greens, kale), garlic, leek, nuts, onion, rocket salad, shallot	Anti-aging Anti-bacterial Anti-inflammatory Antioxidant Anti-platelet Anti-viral Fibrinolytic Protects against CVD Strengthens immune function
• Indoles and Glucosinolates	Cruciferous vegetables (broccoli, Brussels sprouts, cabbage, cauliflower, collard greens, kale), mustard seeds	Blocks & detoxifies carcinogens Blocks tumor growth Limits production of cancer-related hormones
• Isothiocyanates	Cruciferous vegetables (broccoli, Brussels sprouts, cabbage, cauliflower, collard greens, kale)	Antioxidant Blocks tumor growth Detoxifies carcinogens
• Sulforaphane	Broccoli	Cancer chemoprevention Blocks tumor growth (glioma treatment)
Phytic Acid (Inositol)	Bran from corn, oats, rice, rye and wheat, common bean, nuts, peas, soybeans and soy products (edamame, tofu, soy milk)	Anti-cancer (breast & colon) Antioxidant Lowers cholesterol Lowers plasma glucose Lowers plasma insulin Lowers plasma triacylglycerols

	Phytochemical(s)	Plant source	Possible benefits/protection
	Polyphenols (Anthocyanins, Catechin, Curcumin, ECGC, Ellagic acid, Isoflavones, Resveratrol, Quercetin)	Apples, berries, citrus fruits, cocoa, coffee, grapes, green tea, peanuts, soybeans and soy products (edamame, tofu, soy milk), teas whole grains, wine, yams	Anti-cancer Anti-inflammatory Antioxidant Blocks tumor growth Boosts production of detoxifying enzymes Strengthens immune function
	• Anthocyanins	Black rice, blueberries, cherries, chokecherries, grapes, oranges, radishes, red cabbage, red wine	Antioxidant Boosts cognitive function Decreases muscle soreness
Flavanols	• Catechin	Apples, berries, grapes, teas	Alzheimer's disease Anti-bacterial Anti-cancer Anti-caries Antioxidant Diabetes Protects and preserves brain cell structure Regulates metabolism
Flavanols	• Epigallocatechin Gallate (EGCG)	Green tea	Anti-aging Anti-cancer (gastric and pancreatic) Diabetes
Isoflavonoids	• Curcumin	Cumin, turmeric	Alzheimer's disease Anti-aging Anti-bacterial Anti-cancer (adrenal, brain, colorectal, oral, ovarian) Anti-fungal Anti-inflammatory Antioxidant Anti-spasmatic Anti-viral Blocks tumor growth Cancer chemoprevention Detoxifying agent Eases symptoms of ulcerative colitis Hepato-protective Prevents obesity
Flavanols	• Quercetin	Apples (near the skin), berries, brassica vegetables, broccoli, capers, gingko biloba, grapes, honey, onion (outer most rings and closest to root of red onion), red wine, shallot, tea, tomatoes	Alzheimer's disease Anti-bacterial Anti-cancer (breast cancer) Anti-inflammatory Antioxidant CVD (reduces LDL oxidation & atherosclerotic lesions) Inhibits lipid peroxidation Prevents obesity Psychostimulant Reduces blood pressure or hypertension Reduces capillary permeability

	Phytochemical(s)	Plant source	Possible benefits/protection
	• Ellagic Acid	Grapes, strawberries, walnuts	Anti-bacterial Antioxidant Protects against CVD
	• Isoflavones	Soybeans and soy products (edamame, tofu, soy milk, etc.)	Antioxidant Blocks tumor growth Limits production of cancer-related hormones Lowers cholesterol Protects against CVD Reduces risk of osteoporosis Relieves menopausal symptoms
Stilbenes	• Resveratrol	Bilberries, blueberries, cocoa, cranberries, grapes, peanuts, pistachios	Anti-apoptotic Anti-cancer Anti-inflammatory Antioxidant Anti-platelet Blocks tumor proliferation Blood glucose lowering Cancer chemoprevention Prevents endometriosis Positive influence on blood lipid profile Protects against CVD Regulates metabolism
	Terpenes	Algae, black pepper, celery seeds, cherries, cinnamon, citrus fruit peel, cloves, coffee, ginger, mosses, oregano, rosemary, sage	Anti-cancer (breast) Anti-inflammatory Anti-microbial Antioxidant Anti-spasmodic Anti-viral Limits production of cancer-related hormones Protects cells from becoming cancerous Reduces blood pressure or hypertension Slows cancer cell growth Strengthens immune function

*Eggs may offer lutein in a form that's more accessible (fat in yolk may improve absorption)

Sources:[33,109,151,252–259]

Spice it Up!

Don't forget about herbs and spices, which can have even more concentrated levels of phytochemicals, boosting your plant-based power. For example, one study showed that 2 tablespoons of dried basil have twice as much antioxidant power as a cup of green grapes and three times as much as a cup of cooked carrots.[260,261] Always top your plant-based proteins and foods with herbs and spices – nature's most potent antioxidants!

Color Benefits and Phytochemicals

You've heard it before, but we'll say it again, embrace every color in your diet! The colors of different foods are associated with certain phytochemicals. Here's a breakdown of some of the phytochemicals associated with each color, with plant-based examples in each category.

Green – contain the antioxidant lutein which is important for our eye, skin, and heart health. Examples of foods that contain lutein include broccoli, spinach, cucumbers, leafy greens, artichokes, green peppers, green beans, celery, okra, asparagus, kiwi, grapes, apples, limes, and honeydew.[262] Green peas and soybeans also have lutein, and are also good plant-based protein options.[263,264]

Red – contain the antioxidants lycopene and anthocyanin, which are anti-inflammatory and integral in heart health and memory. They may also decrease your risk of developing cancer. Examples include tomatoes, red peppers, red onions, and beets. For a protein source, consider pinto or kidney beans.[262,265]

Yellow and orange – have vitamin C, as well as carotenoids and bioflavonoids, two important antioxidants. These phytochemicals are important for heart and eye health, may decrease the progression of arthritis, and reduce your risk of developing certain cancers, including lung, stomach, bladder, and breast. They are also important for our immune system. Think of pumpkin, yellow and orange peppers, carrots, squash, sweet potatoes, nectarines, oranges, and cantaloupe.[262] Cornmeal and buckwheat are a couple of sources that also contain protein.[266,267]

Purple – are rich in flavonoids, which can help reduce your risk of developing heart disease and cancer, as well as decrease memory loss. Foods in this category include eggplant, purple cabbage, purple asparagus, and plums.[262] Black-eyed peas contain flavonoids in addition to plant-based protein.[268]

White and tan colored beans and legumes contain isoflavones, which have been associated with decreased risk of breast cancer among women and prostate cancer among men. They also function as antioxidants and may decrease the risk of diabetes and cancer, reduce inflammation, and protect our neurons. Soybeans are the best source of isoflavones. Foods such as tofu, tempeh, miso, and soymilk are both high in isoflavones and plant-based protein.[269] White and brown foods also contain polyphenols, which are important for reducing the risk of developing heart disease, osteoporosis, certain types of cancers, and diabetes. Polyphenols are also important for brain health. Cloves, star anise, cocoa powder, and celery seeds are examples of foods high in polyphenols. Flaxseeds, wheat, and other whole grains, lentils, and soy products contain protein in addition to polyphenols.[267,270,271]

Phytonutrients and Sports Nutrition

Some key phytonutrients studied specifically in regard to athletic performance include resveratrol, quercetin (a flavonoid), EGCG (a flavonoid - polyphenol), and curcumin. Some proposed benefits of these compounds are a decrease in reactive oxygen species and a decrease in inflammation, with improved mitochondrial function and improved mental stimulation.[59]

- resveratrol – found in grapes, peanuts, cocoa
- quercetin – found in onions, broccoli, apples (near the skin)[272]
- EGCG (epigallocatechin gallate) – found in green tea
  - Be cautious with green tea supplements, as many do not contain the stated amount of EGCG on the label. Green tea can also interfere with many medications.
- curcumin – found in turmeric

Boosting Phytonutrients

If you're eating a plant-based diet in a variety of colors, it's going to be naturally high in "fight-o-nutrients!" Remember, the intake in color diversity needs to be consistent – one day a week at one meal isn't the solution. Only 12.2% of adults meet the daily fruit intake recommendation and only 9.3% of adults meet the daily vegetable recommendation.[273] A little bit of planning can go a long way. Aim for at least five colors per day. Get the minimum of 1.5-2 cups of fruits per day and 2-3 cups of vegetables per day – then work your way up! Make a list of five new plant-based foods and their corresponding color that you commit to trying this month. Scroll through the phytochemical table and review the benefits that match your health goals. Then create a food list and place it on your refrigerator or schedule some grocery shopping into your calendar. Make this an action item, rather than a disappearing intention.

NUTRITION TIP

Cocoa Powder – a rich and delicious plant-based food.

Adding cocoa powder to dishes can be a good source of magnesium and help with chocolate cravings. It's good for lung health and prevents insulin resistance – and it sure does make your food taste good!

What's the difference between cacao and cocoa?

Both originate from the cacao plant and undergo similar processing, including fermentation, drying, and grinding.[274] However, raw cacao skips the roasting step unlike its cocoa counterpart and is cold pressed to separate the fat from the cacao.[275] Cocoa is packed with flavonoids. Heating diminishes the flavonoid and antioxidant content, making cacao a slightly better choice.[62,276] Flavonoids are important for arterial health and may lower oxidative stress, which occurs naturally as a result of exercise. Both are rich in magnesium and fiber. Cocoa powder can be part of a healthy plant diet and help give your meals a flavor boost when training. We've pulled together a quick nutrient comparison of cocoa and cacao powders to show you their differences side by side in table 5.3.[62]

5.3 - Nutrition Comparison of Cacao and Cocoa for 2 Tablespoons	Cacao	Cocoa
Calories	40	40
Protein (g)	2	2
Fat (g)	0	1
Carbs (g)	6	6
Fiber (g)	4	4
Calcium (mg)	0	0
Iron (mg)	1.5	1.5
Magnesium (mg)	64	54
Potassium (mg)	200	165

To bring everything back full circle, here is a chart **(5.4 - Nutrient Profiles of Plant-Based and Animal Proteins for 100 Calories on pages 137-139)** with different types of protein-rich foods – from both plant and animal sources. Take time to glance over this and see if you can notice any big differences between the two categories. (Hint: fiber, saturated fat, and phytochemicals).

Food	Amt.	Pro (g)	Carb (g)	Fiber (g)	Fat (g)	Unsat fat (g)	Sat fat (g)	Phytonutrients[109]
Tofu, firm	4½ oz.	12	3	2	5	5	0	Isoflavones
Tempeh	⅓ cup.	11	4	4	6	4	1	Isoflavones
Green peas	¾ cup	7	19	7	0	0	0	Lutein
Black beans	½ cup	7	20	8	0	0	0	Anthocyanin
Kidney beans	½ cup	7	19	6	0	0	0	Lycopene, Anthocyanin
Lentils	½ cup	8	18	7	0	0	0	Polyphenols
Walnuts	8 halves	3	2	1	11	10	1	Flavonoids including flavones, flavonols, proanthocyanidins, and anthocyanidins; phytosterols; Tannins including ellagitannins; Syringic acid: Tocopherols
Almonds	14 almonds	4	4	3	10	9	1	Flavonoids, including catechins, flavonols and flavonones in their aglycone and glycoside forms
Peanuts	2 Tbsp.	5	3	1	9	7.5	1.5	Resveratrol
Quinoa	½ cup, cooked	4	20	3	2	1	0	Flavonoids
Farro	⅓ cup, cooked	4	19	2	1	1	0	Lutein (Carotenoids)
Brown rice	½ cup, cooked	2	23	2	1	0	0	Phenolic acids

5.4 - Nutrient Profiles of Plant-Based and Animal Proteins for 100 Calories

5.4 - Nutrient Profiles of Plant-Based and Animal Proteins for 100 Calories (Continued)

Food	Amt.	Pro (g)	Carb (g)	Fiber (g)	Fat (g)	Unsat fat (g)	Sat fat (g)	Phytonutrients[109]
Oats	⅔ cup, cooked	4	17	2	2	1	0	Avenanthramides, a type of phenolic compounds found only in oats β -Glucan in oat bran
Amaranth	⅓ cup, cooked	4	18	2	2	1	0	Betalains
Hemp seeds	1¾ Tbsp.	6	1	1	9	8	1	Cannabinoids, Terpenes and Phenolic compounds
Chia seeds	1¾ Tbsp.	4	9	7	7	6	1	Phenolic compounds
Egg (80 kcal)	I XL egg	7	0	0	5	3	2	Lutein, zeaxanthin
Full fat Greek yogurt	⅓ cup	9	4	0	5	3	2	
0% Greek yogurt	⅔ cup	17	6	0	1	0	0	
Part-skim Mozzarella cheese	1¼ oz.	9	1	0	6	2	4	
Cheddar cheese, reduced fat	1 oz.	9	1	0	6	2	4	

Food	Amt.	Pro (g)	Carb (g)	Fiber (g)	Fat (g)	Unsat fat (g)	Sat fat (g)	Phytonutrients[109]
Full-fat milk	⅔ cup	5	8	0	5	2	3	
Low-fat milk	1 cup	8	12	0	2	1	1	
Kefir, plain	¾ cup	9	12	0	2	1	2	
Salmon, cooked	2 oz.	15	0	0	4	3	1	
Tuna, light, in water	3 oz.	22	0	0	1	0	0	
Sardines	⅓ cup	12	0	0	6	4	1	
Turkey, light meat	2½ oz.	21	0	0	1	1	0	
Turkey, dark meat	2 oz.	16	0	0	3	2	1	
Chicken breast w/ skin	1½ oz.	15	0	0	4	2	1	
Chicken breast w/o skin	2 oz.	19	0	0	2	1	0	
Beef, 80% lean	1½ oz.	11	0	0	8	4	3	
Beef, 95% lean	2 oz.	15	0	0	4	2	2	

Part 6:
SUPPLEMENTS AND ERGOGENIC AIDS

Ergogenic Aids

T
O START OFF, WHAT IS an ergogenic aid? Companies design these with the aim to increase physical power, mental strength or mechanical edge. Athletes take them with the intent of enhancing performance and recovery, improving or maintaining health, increasing energy, compensating for a perceived lack of a nutrient, supporting immunity, or manipulating body composition. It is something that is taken to improve exercise performance and/or enhance training adaptations – think physical power, mental strength or mechanical edge.[277]

Keep in mind that even if a supplement is derived from a natural ingredient or product, this does not necessarily mean that it is safe or effective. There are many supplements on the market that "promote weight loss" or "boost your workout" such as fat burners or pre-workout supplements. Many of these contain "proprietary blends" of various ingredients, which we've told you are something to look out for – especially if you are a competitive athlete that may be tested for specific banned substances!

In addition, many popular nutrient supplements taken by athletes don't provide a performance or health benefit, and may even be detrimental. Consuming an excess of some essential nutrients can be toxic and potentially reduce performance – having an ergolytic, or impairing, effect. Sometimes these surpluses can add up unknowingly, such as if you're eating energy bars that have added vitamins and minerals in addition to your supplemented protein shakes or multivitamin and mineral.

Before taking a supplement consider these points:

- safety and possible hidden ingredients
- efficacy, dosage, potency
- appropriateness for one's sports
- cost
- anti-doping regulations
- claims noted on packaging

- placebo – your potential personal bias
- manufacturing origin, USA or overseas

Having to sift through the research to know what is safe and understand the risk-benefit is no easy task, plus it can be very time-consuming! Understanding there is potential harm to your health and performance is critical. Just because you're reading about something everywhere online, and your friends and teammates are taking it, doesn't mean it's safe or right for you! Utilize the resources we provide in the next section, and if possible, work with a dietitian.[78]

You could be producing some very expensive urine or damaging your kidneys.

While something as simple as carbohydrates from food can be seen as an ergogenic aid (when timed around exercise), many other nutrients and ingredients fall under the supplement umbrella. This is also influenced by the form that they come in and what they are mixed with. As you'll learn with this protein powder review, make sure you're doing your homework when it comes time to purchase a new product. While we aren't going to tackle all of the ergogenic aids you've probably heard about, there are a few that we thought were worth the spotlight.[278]

Safety First with Supplements – How to Make Good Purchases

As a quick note before we dive into the supplement space, keep in mind that most dietitians believe in the "food first" mentality. Supplements cannot make up for a poor diet. In addition, nutrients work together in the body, which we like to call a synergistic relationship. Food is more than the sum of its individual nutrients, and how your body responds to eating food versus supplements can vary. For example, if you're taking vitamins A, D, E, or K, they need fat to be taken up by the body, which is why they're considered the fat-soluble vitamins. Phytonutrients also work together, although they're often studied in isolation, which makes it difficult to assess how they impact the body as a whole. For example, there are over 600 types of carotenoids, but we typically only hear about beta-carotene.

As you'll learn in the next few pages, the supplement industry has a lot of loopholes and potential risks for you as an athlete. If you choose whole foods, you are assuring that you are getting the fuel and nutrients your body needs to stay healthy and perform at your best. However, we all know there are times when individual nutrients are needed or recommended; for example, vitamin D if blood levels are low. There may be times when an athlete has an acute injury with pain and inflammation and wants a natural alternative to ibuprofen because of stomach issues. And there are those times, when you really, just really, want a protein shake! Also, many athletes have extremely high daily caloric needs from hours of exercise each day, and for those athletes, it can be difficult to meet needs via food alone. Believe it or not, people get tired of chewing (and eating!). Let's take a look at the key things you should consider before purchasing anything "protein-powder" related.

Since nearly all protein powders fall under the supplement umbrella, the FDA does not test these products, or much less, even review the products for their safety and effectiveness before they are available for you to purchase.[279] Regulatory agencies will get involved if an adverse event occurs that is suspected to be linked to an adulterated supplement. As a consumer, it can be difficult to know if the label is accurate and if the associated claims listed on the label are sound. As a competitive athlete, it can also be frustrating to figure out if a product meets your sport's league regulations.

The good news is that in mid-February 2019, FDA Commissioner Scott Gottlieb, M.D. posted a statement about new regulations and oversight for supplements. This is supposedly the biggest change within the past 25 years. One of the FDA's main goals is to make sure the public has access to safe and lawful supplements. The steps they plan to take "include communicating to the public as soon as possible when there is a concern about a dietary supplement on the market, ensuring that our regulatory framework is flexible enough to adequately evaluate product safety while also promoting innovation, continuing to work closely with our industry partners, developing new enforcement strategies and continuing to engage in a public dialogue to get valuable feedback from dietary supplement stakeholders."[280]

Manufacturing procedures add to the uncertainty and increase the risk of contamination.[281] Extracting protein isolates from their original food source can also be an unreliable process. In a study that analyzed protein extraction methods, researchers found varying degrees of heavy metals and other impurities in the resulting protein powders. Not only does this call safety into question, but it also may influence its effect on muscle growth.[282] Again, since these supplements do not have standardized regulations beyond manufacturers' promises of safety, as a consumer, it is important to take matters into your own hands to make an informed decision. Consumer Lab is an independent, third-party verification company that evaluates dietary supplements based on the accuracy of their labels and the integrity of their contents. In 132 popular protein powders from 52 brands, a majority contained detectable amounts of arsenic (83.5%), cadmium (73.7%) lead (71.4%), Bisphenol A (BPA) (55%), and mercury (28.6%).[283] Many of these powders also had levels of contaminants that exceed safe limits. Plant protein powders did not fare any better.[284] Consumer Lab is one of many third-party certifiers who test products to ensure their safety and effectiveness. Let's take a look at a few others that you should keep an eye out for.

Is it Certified?

While Consumer Lab is an excellent resource, if you can't find what you're looking for, the website Supplement OWL also provides product recommendations. There are also some other ways to evaluate the quality of supplements to show the product contains what's listed on the label and that it has been tested for banned substances. Competitive athletes don't want a positive drug test due to label inaccuracies – or for any reason! Plus, there are seals you can look for directly on the labels of the supplements you are purchasing. Just know that even if something is labeled as safe, but it ends up being contaminated, the athlete will be held 100% accountable. This is one key reason why we say it's best to meet your protein needs from foods! Here's your breakdown:

NSF Certified for Sport[285]

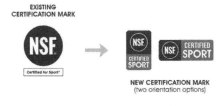

EXISTING
CERTIFICATION MARK

NEW CERTIFICATION MARK
(two orientation options)

NSF Certified for Sport is a trusted source to ensure your supplements do not contain athletic organization-banned substances. It is recognized by the Major League Baseball (MLB), National Hockey League (NHL), Professional Golfers' Association (PGA), National Football League (NFL), and other professional sports leagues. This certification is the gold standard in the sports world. Its stringent testing procedures also include a verification that the label is an accurate representation of the product, a test to make sure it is free of contaminants and follows standard Good Manufacturing Practices (GMP). The mark was recently updated, so so keep an eye out for all three.

Informed Sport[286]

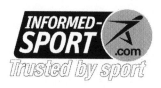

Informed Sport is another third-party tester that checks for the World Anti-Doping Agency's banned substances, ensures quality from raw material through final processing, compares label to contents, and performs routine inspections on their certified partners.

Informed Choice[287]

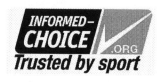

Although this may not be ideal for competitive athletes, it's another third-party certification. Informed Choice is the sister company to Informed Sport. Their testing standards are similar, but the frequency differs. Informed Choice conducts monthly assessments after a product has hit the shelves, while Informed Sport checks every batch before it is released to the public.

USP[288]

U.S. Pharmacopeia Convention (USP) is typically found on many vitamin and mineral products. USP ensures that products contain the amount and strength of the ingredients listed on the label and that they do not contain any unwanted extras (i.e., heavy metals, pesticides, etc.). The most common products tested are vitamin and mineral supplements.

CONSUMER BEWARE

Keep an eye out for "proprietary blend" on the Supplement Facts panel. You typically want to avoid these because they don't list the exact ingredients and amounts.

Do You Need a Protein Shake?

You've likely seen many different protein shakes and powders on the store shelves and heard how important they are for your workout. Do you find yourself wondering if you actually need the extra protein? Do you have a hard time choosing which one is best? Here are the basics so you can navigate the protein powder world with ease.

Research has shown that once protein needs are achieved, additional supplementation does not lead to significantly greater muscle growth.[289,290] Now that you've determined your needs, you may feel that it is challenging to meet them based on your busy schedule, or your usual dietary pattern. Occasionally if you lift later in the day, you may be too beat to eat a meal, or not that hungry, and a ready-made salad and a protein shake are the perfect meal for that day. Even though minimally processed whole foods are always the best source of nutrition, a supplemental protein powder shake could be an option worth exploring if you find you aren't quite reaching your target.

Animal-Based Protein Powder Overview

Animal-derived proteins are generally better absorbed in the body than plant-based proteins. However, there is more to good nutrition than just biological value. Plus, you can add in a few more grams of plant protein to help make up the difference in amino acids, like leucine. Plant-based proteins are usually sufficient for most individuals, but if you are struggling to see results, perhaps exploring a few animal-based options could help. Or, you can try creating an animal to plant ratio that works for you. Whey, casein, and egg are common protein powders on the market. Each has unique proposed benefits. Let's dive in!

Whey

Whey is the most widespread type of protein powder sold in stores. It is available as a concentrate, isolate, or hydrolysate. Concentrate is simply whey with water removed and is typically 70-80% protein. Isolate goes a step further and removes most lactose, fat, and cholesterol, which is why it is typically 90% or higher in protein by weight. Hydrolysate breaks down the protein into easily digested amino acids for easier absorption, and it can be made from whey protein concentrate or isolate. All three types are similar in their high bioavailability and effectiveness in stimulating muscle protein synthesis.[284,291,292]

- 1 ounce of whey protein isolate = 27 grams of protein and 2.9 grams of leucine

Casein

Casein is a slower digesting milk-based protein powder. It is less bioavailable than whey and soy, but due to its prolonged digestion, researchers believe that taking casein at night may combat protein catabolism during sleep. However, study results have been mixed.[284]

- 1 ounce of micellar casein = 26 grams of protein and 2.4 grams of leucine[293]

Egg

Egg white protein powder has limited scientific research in terms of muscle protein synthesis. One study showed that it had sufficient leucine to promote muscle protein synthesis. When compared to whey, soy, and wheat, it was second best to whey in its muscle building abilities. Instead of buying egg powder, just work in more eggs or egg whites into your plant-based meals. For example, bean burgers made with egg whites, savory oatmeal with eggs, or a bean and hardboiled egg salad.

- 1 ounce of egg white protein = 25 grams of protein and 2.3 grams of leucine[294]

Collagen

Collagen is a main structural protein in skin, tendons, ligaments, and other connective tissues. There are over ten types of collagen all originating from animal sources, but two are the most abundant that you will see in many products: Type 1 (hydrolyzed) and Type 2 (undenatured). You'll see both types in sports nutrition but may see more of Type 2. It can be taken for a variety of reasons: joint mobility, knee extension, or osteoarthritis.[295,296] The IOC consensus statement on dietary supplements and high-performance athletes states that supplements appear to be low risk. Although little data is available, it does show increased collagen production and possible decreased pain.

Collagen & Bone Broth

Collagen and bone broth powder have been trending in the wellness and sports nutrition space, but the two shouldn't be confused. Bone broth contains collagen, but depending on the product, there are different amounts of collagen. Beef bone broth has been found to have more collagen than chicken bone broth.[284] However, because of the various levels in bone broth, and the unspecified amounts of each type, if you are trying to focus on collagen itself, explore collagen supplements. There has also been some talk about high lead levels in bone broth due to the leaching of lead from bones.[297] However, Consumer Lab testing of popular bone broth products didn't find any contaminated products with levels that were above the heavy metal threshold.

Collagen is a component of gelatin. You will most likely see collagen as collagen peptides, which means that gelatin has been taken and processed so that it is further broken down and easier to digest. While most popular collagen products come from land animals and birds, there are also collagen supplements that come from marine vertebrates and invertebrates, and fish. The latter sources are commonly referred to as marine collagen.[298] This is a good alternative for pesco-vegetarians.

Proponents of this supplement cite its ability to reduce joint pain in adults and athletes, and benefit hair, improve skin elasticity and strengthen nails.[299,300] Some even claim it can reduce cellulite and wrinkles.[301,302]

In the sports space, collagen has been used primarily for recovery and joint issues. Its close relative, gelatin, is paired with vitamin C to promote collagen synthesis for rehab purposes. Amounts of 5-15 grams of gelatin with 50 milligrams of vitamin C (the more taken in this range, the more the benefit) taken one hour before training is a typical dose.[89,303,304] However, if you just stick with collagen, 10 grams of collagen hydrolysate is recommended.[89] Collagen also showed promising results for athletes looking for more ankle stability.[305] In older adults, studies have demonstrated its effectiveness against age-related muscle mass loss, despite collagen's low leucine content.[306,307]

But how does it stack up for muscle building? The first thing to remember is that collagen isn't considered a complete protein – it is lacking one of the nine essential amino acids, tryptophan, and many of its amino acids are in much greater abundance than others. It is also low in methionine. To put the importance of this in perspective, it scores 0.0 on DIAAS, making it a low-quality protein.[48] Its leucine content is quite low as well – it would take about 75 grams of collagen to get 2 grams of leucine. Most serving sizes of collagen on popular products are 10-20 grams. If you're looking to gain muscle, consider it as an add-on to other protein at your meal.

- 1 ounce of collagen peptides = 30 grams of protein and 0.8 grams of leucine (*note that a typical serving is 20 grams)[307]

Plant Protein Powder Overview

"Amino acid profiles largely differed among plant-based proteins with leucine contents ranging from 5.1% for hemp to 13.5% for corn protein, compared to 9.0% for milk, 7.0% for egg, and 7.6% for muscle protein."[308] This shows that plant-based proteins can hold their own against animal proteins! See more on plant protein's amino acid breakdown on MelissasHealthyLiving.com. There are four sources of plant protein powder most often seen on the shelves. Here is a breakdown:

Pea

Pea protein has recently become much more popular in the supplement space. One study compared whey and pea protein supplements and found comparable increases in muscle thickness from participants in both groups, so pea protein serves as a good substitute for those who want an alternative to whey.[309] It is important to note that the leucine content of the pea protein used was 6.4 grams. While this was less than the 8.6 grams in the whey protein, it was still well over the 2-3 grams threshold for muscle protein synthesis. Some people don't like the taste of 100% pea, which is one reason you often see blends.

- 1 ounce of pea powder = 27 grams of protein and 2.7 grams of leucine[310]

Soy

Soy is a complete protein and has a digestibility score that rivals milk-based proteins, which is why it is often compared against whey. Though soy protein is a complete protein, it only has small amounts of methionine.[284] The research is mixed on its effect on protein synthesis and athletic performance. Some studies show comparable or improved muscle protein synthesis when compared to the milk proteins whey and casein. In short-term studies, soy has also been seen to be as effective as casein – the protein that makes up about 80% of milk.[311] Additionally, a recent meta-analysis looking at nine different long-term studies comparing soy and animal protein supplementation (whey, beef, milk, or dairy) with resistance exercise training found that both groups had significant gains in strength, and there were no differences between the soy and whey groups.[311] Despite these results, some studies suggest soy protein is inferior. This may seem conflicting, however, if you're making progress towards your body composition goals, then you're likely meeting your protein needs.[290,312] In general once you meet your determined protein needs, excess protein intake won't provide any additional benefit. Bottom line: meet your protein needs, don't exceed them, then monitor your workout, and evaluate your results.

- 1 ounce of soy protein isolate = 25 grams of protein and 1.9 grams of leucine[62]

Rice

Rice protein is a hypoallergenic option with sufficient amounts of the amino acid, leucine, comparable to whey protein isolate. Leucine is particularly important in promoting muscle protein synthesis.[313] The main thing to keep an eye out for with rice protein powders is to make sure you are using a supplement from a reliable source because many rice-derived products are contaminated with arsenic.[284]

- 1 ounce of rice powder = 25 grams of protein and 2.1 grams of leucine[314]

Hemp

Hemp protein brings unique nutritional components to a protein shake with regards to its high antioxidant and fiber content. For general comparison, hemp protein has a lower percentage of BCAAs than whey and soy, but higher than rice and egg protein.[311] For competitive collegiate or professional athletes, or those who are drug tested, it is typically encouraged not to consume hemp, since it is harvested from the hemp plant *Cannabis sativa.* Consuming hemp protein increases the risk of a positive drug test due to traces of THC, even if the product claims that it doesn't contain THC.

- 1 ounce of hemp powder = 15 grams of protein and 0.8 grams of leucine[62]

What Else Is in the Bottle?

Soy, rice, pea, and hemp are commonly used as the base of plant-based protein supplements. Sometimes they are sold individually, but more often they are sold as a proprietary blend where the exact ratio of the mixture is unspecified. This may be done to achieve a more balanced amino acid profile and taste; however, in some cases, it can hinder transparency for the consumer. On occasion, a label may separately indicate a list of the exact amounts of each amino acid, which can help an athlete make an informed decision based on their needs. But given the varied nature of blended products, it makes it difficult to conduct research on its effectiveness and create mass recommendations for the public. If you are uncertain about the dosing, consult with your RDN.

Other ingredients such as sweeteners, fiber, caffeine, creatine, individual amino acids, vitamins, and minerals are also commonly added to supplements. These additives are often hidden in fine print on the label or within trademarked blends, which do not legally require manufacturers to list exact amounts of each addition.[281] Keep an eye out for these and always be your own detective when buying supplements!

Your Plant Protein Takeaways

Now that you're more familiar with all that protein powder can do (or not do), you can decide how it may fit into your typical eating pattern. It is also important to remember that you'll likely be mixing this protein powder with something else – boosting the nutrient profile (and taste!). While many people like to mix their protein powder into a smoothie, some like to just mix it with a liquid for easy on-the-go consumption. Anytime you mix your powder with something else, be aware of the nutrition composition of the liquid (i.e., water, milk, juice, etc.) and/or the foods you're adding to make sure you're staying on track with your overall needs!

From this closer look at plant and animal-based protein powders, you can see that they have many different characteristics and that some are better than others. They also can vary quite a bit in their flavor profile. Here are a few key takeaways:

- keep the leucine amount in mind if you have certain body composition goals
- understand that there is a benefit to some plant-protein mixes to achieve a desirable amino acid profile
- both animal and plant-based protein powders can help you meet your needs

Head to MelissasHealthyLiving.com for brand recommendations and a breakdown of nutrition facts, special features, additives, and third-party certifications! Join the newsletter for updates for helpful product recommendations.

Caffeine

Caffeine is a food ingredient, dietary supplement, and FDA-approved drug naturally found in a variety of plant foods such as coffee, green and black tea, and cocoa.[84] Caffeine stimulates the central nervous system (heart function, blood circulation, and the release of epinephrine (adrenaline)), and has been suspected to influence athletic performance.[78]

The International Olympic Committee (IOC) shows strong evidence regarding caffeine as an ergogenic aid among athletes. Still, it is important to consider that a consumer's response to caffeine is personal and may vary based on a variety of factors, such as diet, health status (and/or body composition) and genetics. As with any food or safe supplement caffeine's effect should be evaluated during training prior to use in competition!

How does it work?
- Caffeine increases the release of endorphins, reduces perceived fatigue, and increases alertness, which may improve simple reaction time.[89]
- Caffeine may raise serum free fatty acid (FFA) levels at rest just before exercise. The current belief is that this will enhance the metabolism of FFA, while decreasing the need for glycogen, and may ultimately increase the length of time until fatigue during exercise.[84]
- Current data suggest that caffeine ingestion prior to exercise will induce a glycogen-sparing effect and can also aid carbohydrate uptake post-exercise.

Is it safe?
- At the proper doses, caffeine consumption is safe.
- Caffeine doses of ≥9 milligrams per kilogram of body weight are often accompanied by undesirable side effects such as anxiety, nausea, shakiness, elevated heart rate and/or insomnia. Very large doses (up to 30 grams) can be dangerous and potentially fatal.[89]
- Athletes with hypertension, impaired kidney function, or those who are sensitive to caffeine should consume with caution.
- A caffeine-specific gene, CYP1A2, controls how fast or slow we metabolize caffeine, which is why certain people may respond much more (or less) to the same dose. This is why it's important to experiment with the dose that works best for you.
- Literature does not confirm caffeine-related diuresis during exercise or changes in fluid balance that would harm performance.

How should it be consumed?

- Caffeine may be consumed in various forms, such as sports gels/confectionery, energy drinks, bars and other beverages (coffee, tea, cocoa).
- It is generally recommended to take 3-6 milligrams of caffeine per kilogram body weight about 50-60 minutes before exercise.[89] This is equivalent to about 1-3 cups of coffee for a 150-pound person.
- Sports scientists suspect consuming caffeine with carbohydrate may offer synergistic benefits for prolonged, high-intensity, intermittent activity.[84]
- The National Collegiate Athletic Association (NCAA) considers caffeine a banned substance if urine concentrations are >15 micrograms of caffeine/mL of urine. This is equal to about 500 milligrams (6-8 cups of coffee) 2-3 hours before the event.[315]

6.1 - Caffeine in Select Beverages

Food or beverage	Amount (oz.)	Caffeine content (mg)
Brewed coffee, generic Starbucks (Dark, Blonde) Dunkin' Donuts	8 16 (grande) 14 (med)	75-165 260, 360 164
Cold brew, Starbucks	16	205
Decaffeinated coffee, generic	6	2
Brewed tea, black Green Decaffeinated black	8	40-70 25-40 2
Snapple	16	22
Mountain Dew	12	54
Energy drink, generic Rockstar Red Bull 5-hr Energy	8 8 8.4 1.9	77 80 75 200

Sources:[316–318]

For a comprehensive list of caffeine sources, see Caffeine Chart on MelissasHealthyLiving.com.

Who is it most effective for?

- Individuals practicing endurance and high-intensity activity
- Individuals engaging in short term exercise and/or repeated sprint tasks

Key Takeaway: Caffeine, consumed at a low-to-moderate dose of roughly 3-6 milligrams per kilogram of body weight, may improve performance for healthy athletes practicing aerobic and anaerobic exercise.[89]

Creatine

 Creatine is a nitrogen-containing compound that is naturally occurring in animal muscle and synthesized by the body.[89] Since creatine is not banned by major organizations (ie. NCAA, IOC), many collegiate and professional sports teams are prevalent users. Research supports a positive ergogenic effect of creatine supplementation in certain exercise endeavors, primarily characterized by repetitive, high-intensity exercise bouts with brief recovery periods.

How does it work?
- Appropriate creatine loading protocols will increase total muscle creatine, which includes free creatine and phosphocreatine. This is often accompanied by a small increase in body mass of 0.6-1 kilograms of body weight.[78,89]
- The ergogenic theory is that increasing creatine phosphate in the muscle will enhance the ATP-PCr energy system.
  - Increased muscle creatine will help resynthesize creatine phosphate to provide more substrate for generating ATP (energy) to help maintain quick explosive movements (such as sprinting) at a high intensity.
- Creatine supplementation may enhance the recovery process and help users maintain lean body mass during periods of injury or immobilization.[89]
- Creatine may offer potential antioxidant and anti-inflammatory benefits.[89]

Is it safe?
- Many studies show it is safe for long-term use of up the four or five years when consumers follow a proper protocol.[89,319]
- It may lead to dehydration and muscle cramps, so a proper fluid strategy is important.
- Occasionally it may cause gastrointestinal (GI) discomfort, such as diarrhea, upset stomach, and belching; further dividing the dose may help with GI tolerance.[78,320]
- Individuals with impaired kidney function should take caution.[320]

- Creatine supplementation may make it more difficult for weight-control athletes to lose weight for competition.

How much should you consume?

- Creatine monohydrate (powder) is the best form. Keep this in mind, as many products do not contain the appropriate form. Work with a sports dietitian if you're considering supplementation.[78]
- Creatine supplementation typically involves a loading phase, and a maintenance phase:[57,321]
    - *Loading phase:* 5 grams creatine monohydrate (~0.3 grams of creatine/kilogram body weight) 4 times a day for 5-7 days (*Loading is unnecessary unless you have limited time before competition)
    - *Maintenance phase:* 3-5 grams per day over 4 weeks or the duration of your supplement protocol. Start this about a month out from competition.
- Combining creatine with simple carbohydrates and protein increases creatine transport into the muscle.[79]

Can you get creatine from food? Of course! In a typical 3-ounce serving, beef has 0.38 grams of creatine, salmon has 0.375 grams, tuna provides 0.34 grams, and herring provides 0.56-0.84 grams.[322]

Who has it been most effective for?
- Those who have the lowest muscle creatine levels before supplementation will increase their levels the most. For example, vegetarians typically have low creatine stores and experience increased uptake of creatine compared to non-vegetarians.[172,319]
- Those engaging in high intensity performance, or stop and go sports that require speed and muscular power.
- Athletes looking to increase lean body mass and strength when combined with resistance training.[319,321]
- Other proposed benefits of creatine include protection of the brain and spinal cord from injury and infarction (notably for athletes at risk of concussion), protection from neurodegenerative diseases, and improved cognitive processing (including during periods of fatigue

or sleep deprivation).[57,89] More research is needed for stronger evidence.

Key Takeaway: Creatine supplementation in a powdered, monohydrate form, taken in appropriate protocols, may improve muscle strength and endurance during high-intensity exercise, preserve lean muscle mass, and shorten recovery periods. As always only use supplements that have been independently tested for safety, with contents that match the labeled dosage.

Carnosine and Creatine with Vegetarian/Vegan Diets

It is also worthwhile to note that carnosine and creatine levels in the muscle are two other amino acid-based compounds that have been studied in vegetarian/vegan power and strength athletes. This population typically has lower levels of both in comparison to athletes who follow an omnivorous diet.[13] This makes sense considering the sources of these compounds are mostly animal based (i.e., from meat, fish, and poultry). Keep in mind that creatine is a non-essential amino acid, so the liver can create it, and the body doesn't rely on getting it from the diet. Carnosine is made from two other amino acids (beta-alanine and histidine), and while histidine is one you need to get from food, this isn't a problem for vegans and vegetarians because soy, nuts, seeds, beans, and whole grains can provide this. While many studies to date find total lower body creatine and lower plasma (in the blood) carnosine in vegetarians and vegans, this hasn't shown a negative impact on performance in comparison to an omnivorous diet.[13]

If you are still concerned about reaching your dietary needs, discuss the need for a supplement with a Registered Dietitian Nutritionist.

Tart Cherry Juice

Tart cherries contain anthocyanins, a type of polyphenol considered a phytonutrient, which acts as an antioxidant and can help reduce inflammation. They also contain an assortment of other health-promoting fight-o-nutrients! Even more, they naturally contain small amounts of melatonin. Tart cherries are not the same as sweet cherries (even though sweet cherries can still be a great phytochemical-rich fruit choice to add to yogurt, smoothies, etc.).

How does it work?

It decreases inflammatory cytokines and/or indirect markers of muscle damage. So essentially, it can help reduce exercise-induced oxidative stress (thanks, antioxidants!) to help your body recover faster. Tart cherries, or tart cherry juice, can also help reduce muscle soreness post-exercise.[89] While more research is needed before we see a consensus on this recommendation, we are seeing it utilized most often in competitive athletes.

How much should you consume?

- 250 to 350 milliliters or 8.5 to 11 ounces (30 milliliters if concentrate) twice daily for 4-5 days before an athletic event or for 2-3 days afterward to promote recovery.
- For someone who is more in the moderately active category, consume 8 ounces right after your workout. It can be part of your recovery snack or meal. Just keep in mind that it does contain carbohydrate and adds in extra liquid calories, so account for this in your daily calorie intake to make sure you aren't consuming extra calories.
- If tart cherry juice is too bitter, you can always add it into a smoothie blended with yogurt, flaxseeds, and other fruit for a great post-workout snack. Check the companion cookbook for some tasty recipes.

Who has it been most effective for?

It can work for a variety of athletes to enhance recovery. Anecdotally, it's often recommended to reduce inflammation or arthritis-like symptoms in sports that are harder on the joints, such as jujitsu, martial arts, or in competitive/elite athletes with intense and extensive training, like marathon runners.

Beet Juice and Nitrates

Beet juice is yet another food that's been studied for its performance enhancement properties. It is packed with anthocyanins, which you probably could have guessed, due to its red-purple color. Beets also have naturally occurring nitrates that have shown to improve performance through their ability to dilate your blood vessels. Other foods that also have naturally occurring nitrates include spinach and celery.[89]

How does it work?

Nitrates are converted to nitric oxide (NO) in the mouth and stomach. Because this conversion starts in the mouth, you should not chew gum after consuming the beet juice – it can decrease its effectiveness. These nitrates decrease blood pressure and allow more blood and oxygen to be delivered to the muscles. This means your body can optimally fuel for longer, and power your workout to delay the feelings of fatigue.

How much should you consume?
- 300-600 milligrams total, or 0.1 millimole of nitrates per kilogram of body weight per day, taken 2-3 hours before exercise.[89] For example, if an athlete wants to calculate their amount needed based on weight, if the individual weighs 140 pounds (63.6 kilograms), the recommendation would be 6.36 millimoles nitrates. An athlete who weighs 180 pounds (81.8 kilograms) would need 8.18 millimoles nitrates.
- Keep in mind that while you can make your own beet juice with a juicer, the concentration of nitrates is lower in these than in many beet juice supplement "shots" on the market.[332] For example, 2 ounces of cooked beets contain 83 milligrams of nitrates, 2 ounces of a commonly sold beet juice contains 121 milligrams, while 2 ounces of a popular beet supplement "shot" contains 333 milligrams.[62,333,334]
- On average, there are 1,459 milligrams of nitrates per 6 cups of cooked sliced beets (1 kilogram), though there is a range of 644-1,800 milligrams of nitrates per kilogram beetroot.[334] This means that you'd have to eat about 1.25 cups of cooked sliced beets to get 300 milligrams of nitrates. It's probably smartest to just stick with the beet shots if you're interested in the benefits day after day (unless you really love beets!).

Who has it been most effective for?
- More research is needed in this area, as evidence is mixed and limited.
- Performance improvements range between 4-25% for time to exhaustion, 1-3% for sport-specific time trials less than 40 minutes, and 3-5% for high intensity intermittent team exercise lasting 12-40 minutes.[89] More evidence is needed for exercise lasting <12 minutes in duration.

Keep in mind that if you begin to consume more beet juice, it may change the color of your urine or stools to have a pink hue – so don't get too alarmed!

NUTRITION FACT

You may have seen nitrates and nitrites on packaged meat and heard a thing or two about how bad they are for you. These nitrates and nitrites aren't naturally occurring and are added to keep the "pinkness" of certain foods, like cured and processed meats. They can contribute to carcinogen synthesis via their contribution to the conversion of nitrates/nitrites to nitrosamines.

How does this differ from the nitrates in beets and other vegetables? Those nitrates are converted to nitric oxide, which is what provides the positive heart and performance effects.

Supplement Snapshots

Caffeinated Herbal Blends

Caffeinated herbal blends including products that contain guarana, kola nut, yerba mate or green tea, should be consumed with caution, as there are safety concerns associated with high doses of caffeine. For example, guarana can be unsafe if taken in excess (doses over 250-300 milligrams per day) for an extended period of time and can be fatal if very high doses are taken.[323] Other caffeine-containing substances, including kola nut and yerba mate, are also unsafe if large or very large doses are taken.[324,325]

Energy Drinks and Shots

These are widely available, with countless brands and types on the market. Despite the multitude of claims on the labels, the ingredients in most drinks proven to be ergogenic are carbohydrate and caffeine. These drinks can also often be a significant source of excess calories, so paying attention to how this contributes to your overall calorie needs is important. Low calorie or sugar-free energy drinks can still improve mental focus, alertness, and exercise performance. However, as these products are freely available to purchase and are often right at the counter when finalizing a purchase, don't be tempted to try one out if you haven't done your research first![326]

Glucosamine and Chondroitin Sulfate

Glucosamine and chondroitin sulfate are frequently taken either separately or in combination in the belief that they maintain joint health and/or have therapeutic benefits for those suffering from arthritic disease. These substances are normally present and synthesized in the body and are concentrated in cartilage. This is why it is suggested these supplements may be 'chondroprotective' - meaning they reduce the breakdown of cartilage. They may also have anti-inflammatory effects and are often marketed to promote healthy joints in individuals who exercise. However, studies offer conflicting evidence on their effectiveness and have mostly been performed on middle-aged and/or older subjects.[327]

For middle-age athletes with joint pain that does not improve with other diet changes, if supplementation is considered, a reasonable dose would be 1,500 milligrams of glucosamine and 1,200 milligrams of chondroitin daily for 2-4 months. If there is therapeutic relief (pain relief and improved mobility), with a safe brand, given its minimal side effects it may be worth trying.[84,327] Research is split on whether each supplement or a combination of the two, reduce severe knee pain among older patients with osteoarthritis.[84] Overall, current studies indicate glucosamine sulfate, alone, may offer the greatest therapeutic benefits.[84]

Consumers may experience mild side effects, such as asthma exacerbation, elevated blood glucose for individuals with diabetes, mild diarrhea and bloating.[84,327] Further research is needed regarding the effectiveness of glucosamine, chondroitin and/or the combination of the two supplements on healthy joints and pain relief.

Beta-Alanine

This amino acid has been studied for its potential to reduce muscle fatigue and increase muscle carnosine content to improve the muscles' buffering capabilities. Similar to creatine, beta-alanine requires a loading phase to reach peak saturation, followed by maintenance doses that can be adjusted based on the training load.[89] There are potential beneficial effects of beta-alanine for high-intensity exercise performance.[89] A mixture of beta-alanine and creatine or sodium bicarbonate for at least a 4-week period may also have small benefits on these short-duration, high-intensity activities, however, further research is needed.[79,278,328] For activities lasting over 10 minutes in duration, little to no benefits on performance have been found.[328] The most common side effect of beta-alanine supplementation is tingling and itchy skin, which can be reduced by using a slow-release formula or splitting up doses.

Sodium Bicarbonate

Commonly known as baking soda, sodium bicarbonate likely has little benefit for exercise durations lasting over 7-10 minutes. There may be only a ~2% performance improvement for high-intensity exercise lasting about 1 minute or for sports with intermittent movement (think of sports such as swimming, sprinting, tennis, or boxing).[89] However, there are conflicting results and variability in response across individuals, with some subjects finding that supplementation led to decreased performance. Consider the pros and cons, specifically paying attention to the potential for gastrointestinal distress. A dose of 0.2-0.4 grams of sodium bicarbonate per kilogram of body weight, taken 60-150 minutes before exercise, may have small benefits on performance if engaging in the type of activity listed above.[89,328]

Arginine

This is an amino acid common in a variety of protein foods and can also be synthesized within the body. Among the limited number of studies that have investigated the effects of arginine supplementation on muscle growth and exercise performance, the results are conflicting, with a lack of evidence to recommend supplementation for ergogenic effects. At this time, it is stated to not be effective for increasing muscle mass or strength.[329] Adverse effects of supplementation include nausea and loose stools.[328]

Glutamine

This non-essential amino acid has the important role of removing excess amino groups from the muscle and delivering them to the kidneys. It is present in high concentration in muscle tissue. There are only a limited number of studies that have investigated glutamine's ergogenic potential, and the results of these studies have not found glutamine supplementation to enhance athletic performance. Glutamine has also been studied for potential exercise-related immune-enhancing functions; however, there is also a lack of evidence in support of glutamine supplementation in this setting.[328]

Branched Chain Amino Acids (BCAA)

This group includes the essential amino acids leucine, isoleucine, and valine. Studies have investigated BCAA supplementation for endurance aerobic exercises, for enhancing muscle mass and several other performance-related measures. While some studies have found positive results, there is currently a limited amount of research and lack of strong evidence to recommend BCAA supplementation for improving athletic performance.[328] In fact, some research has suggested that BCAA supplementation may contribute to nutrition imbalances.[84] A balanced, whole food diet meeting protein needs will be sufficient.[328]

HMB (β-hydroxy-beta-methylbutyrate)

This is a leucine metabolite. HMB is purported to be involved in muscle synthesis and is thought to help repair damaged muscle cells. However, there is a lack of consensus about its ergogenic effects. The current body of research has investigated a variable range of supplement regimens and doses and has included participants with a range of exercise habits and ages. As such, it is difficult to draw conclusions about the ergogenic potential of HMB supplementation for the athlete from this research.[328] An athlete's level of training can also influence the effectiveness.[329] The IOC states that adequate protein from the diet is likely as effective as HMB supplementation.[89]

Banned Substances

Ephedrine

This stimulant is not a permissible ingredient in dietary supplements. Ephedra has been associated with increased risk for adverse reactions compared with other herbs, including heart arrhythmias, myocardial infarction, cardiac arrest, and even sudden death.[330] Pure ephedrine is regulated as a drug, and the FDA allows only very small amounts in over-the-counter drugs such as cold medications.

Although a powerful stimulant, ephedrine by itself has not been shown to consistently enhance exercise performance. Use of ephedrine, ephedra, and ma huang in competition is prohibited by the World Anti-Doping Agency (WADA) and the IOC. Common replacements for ephedra include bitter orange, methylsynephrine, synephrine, and oxilofrine, and these are also banned.[331]

Glycerol

Glycerol is banned by the WADA, so instead of using glycerol, follow the recommended hydration protocols mentioned earlier in this book![78]

A couple of other substances banned by the FDA include androstenedione and dimethylamylamine.[328]

Overall Takeaways

- Beta-alanine supplementation might provide a small increase in performance for high-intensity exercises of short-duration. There are few risks other than skin tingling, which can be bypassed by extended-release capsules.
- Creatine is effective for repetitive high-intensity, short-duration exercise tasks.
- Caffeine may be beneficial for endurance and high-intensity performance through increased alertness and perception. Avoid excess intake of caffeine or caffeinated herbal blends.
- Make sure to read the labels on energy drinks for excess calories and be wary of other added ingredients.
- Sodium bicarbonate supplementation may contribute to a ~2% performance improvement. However, consider the pros and cons, specifically paying attention to the potential for gastrointestinal distress.
- There is no data supporting advantages of oral amino acid supplementation (including arginine and glutamine) over adequate dietary protein intake.[278]
- Branched-chain amino acids do not appear to have an ergogenic effect on exercise performance and may actually lead to nutritional imbalances. Consuming adequate protein from whole foods is sufficient to meet your body's needs.
- Additional research is merited with HMB– consuming adequate protein from food alone should suffice.
- Avoid banned substances, including ephedrine, ephedra, ma huang, bitter orange, methylsynephrine, oxilofrine, synephrine, glycerol,

androstenedione, and dimethylamylamine. If you see these on a label, avoid the product.

- Glucosamine and chondroitin may have benefits for joint health, but further research is needed regarding the effectiveness on athletic performance.

Turmeric and Curcumin

Turmeric is the dried root of the plant Curcuma longa. Have you ever wondered where turmeric gets its beautiful golden color? Well, think no further! It's all from curcuminoids – non-flavonoid polyphenols (powerful phytonutrients) and anti-inflammatory compounds.[109] Curcumin is the most popular of the three curcuminoids, composing about 80% of all three, and is the king of many of the health benefits.[335] Because it is so powerful, you will often see supplements solely composed of curcumin, rather than turmeric.

Fun Fact: Turmeric can actually block the same enzyme cyclooxygenase-2 (COX-2) that Advil blocks. Better yet, you can combine turmeric with your omega-3s, the ultimate anti-inflammatory powerhouses, and it will have an even stronger effect! It's also been shown to effectively help decrease inflammation associated with osteoarthritis of the knee.[336] Anecdotally, I have seen similar results in clients.

Turmeric can be purchased in three main forms:
1. Turmeric Root (the one that looks similar to ginger)
2. Ground Turmeric (a powder you can mix and dust onto your food)
3. Turmeric Supplement (the mighty mix that can have the extract, root, and curcuminoids all in one)

Ways to eat it:
- add the root or ground turmeric to smoothies
- add to lentil, bean, and poultry dishes
- add to hummus, Greek yogurt dips, and dressings
- sprinkle on top of sweet potatoes

See the companion recipe book for more tasty ideas.

SPICY TIP

The type of spice or supplement you purchase, and how you consume it, matters because the bioavailability of the beneficial curcumin compounds found in turmeric can change based on many factors. Most dried herbs and spices lose their antioxidant power after six months.[337] When you open them, date them! You can still use them for flavor, but they won't have the same health benefit.

The good news is there are ways to increase the amount of turmeric your body is able to absorb and metabolize. Two simple ways to do this are:

1. Take it with black pepper (which contains a compound called piperine) – this slows the **elimination time** of turmeric in your body. Your body will hold onto it for longer, which means it can absorb more at that time.
2. Take it with foods containing fats or oils – think of turmeric as a fat lover that binds to the fat in the food you eat. This helps it travel through your body to make itself more available to you.

Recovery from Exercise

In a study done on 20 healthy males who were relatively active, they found a reduction in onset of muscle soreness when given 400 milligrams a day of curcumin (200 milligrams at breakfast, 200 milligrams at dinner) for 4 days (the 2 days prior, the day of, and 1 day post).[338] While more research is needed in this area, it's one study specific to exercise that has promising results.

You'll also get the added benefit of micronutrients. In 1 tablespoon of ground turmeric powder, you will find:[339]

- 2 micrograms folate

- 16 milligrams calcium

- 20 milligrams magnesium

- 5 milligrams iron

- 28 milligrams phosphorus

- 196 milligrams potassium

If you are on other supplements or medications or are breastfeeding or pregnant, it is best to consult with your doctor before use. For more expert advice on supplements, meet with a Registered Dietitian Nutritionist.

Herbs and Spices – Antioxidant Powerhouses that Boost Phytonutrient Power in Your Diet

Basil: Two tablespoons of dried basil have almost the same amount of antioxidants as a tangerine.[260]

Cinnamon: One teaspoon of ground cinnamon has more than twice as many antioxidants as a medium peach.[260]

Parsley: Fresh parsley is surprisingly rich in vitamin A and potassium, and moderately rich in calcium and vitamins C & K.[340]

Oregano: Just 2 teaspoons of oregano dried leaves have twice the antioxidants of a medium size Fuji apple.[341]

Garlic: Contains allicin, another phytonutrient that has anti-bacterial and anti-viral properties.[342,343]

Part 7:
TASTY PLANT-BASED MEAL AND SNACK IDEAS

P LANT-BASED EATING OPENS A WHOLE world of creativity around mealtime. We've touched on so many different grains, legumes, nuts, and seeds that can be the base of any plant-based meal. To tie it all together, check out the companion recipe book for full nutrient breakdowns of many of these items so you have the option to personalize your meals based on certain nutrition needs and taste preferences you have.

Mix-and-Match Bowls and Plates

Who knew meal planning could be this easy? Use this guide to create a nutritionally balanced plant-based, protein-rich meal. Make yourself a plate or throw it all into a bowl and mix it up! To add variety, you can use more than one protein, such as two types of beans or half chickpeas and half tofu. Prepare the ingredients to your preference – stir-fry, roast, or keep them raw; cook with flavor-enhancers like onions, garlic, or ginger; season with your favorite herbs and spices; or serve the meal hot or cold, like a pasta salad. If a bowl or plate doesn't appeal to you, add all of your ingredients into whole grain tortillas and make tacos or wrap into a tortilla to make a burrito.

For a base with a boost of flavor, cook leafy greens and mushrooms with:

- 1 tablespoon water
- 1 teaspoon olive oil
- 1 teaspoon Braggs Liquid Aminos or soy sauce
- 1 tablespoon balsamic vinegar
- 1 crushed garlic clove or ½ teaspoon garlic powder

Then add all the layers!

7.1 - Mix-and-Match Bowls and Plates

Step 1: Choose a vegetable	Step 2: Choose a plant-based protein	Step 3: Choose a grain	Step 4: Top it off	Step 5: Optional dressing/ seasoning
• Asparagus • Avocado • Bell peppers • Broccoli • Brussels sprouts • Carrots • Kale • Mushrooms • Spinach • Tomatoes	• Bean or lentil pasta • Beans (black, kidney, white, pinto) • Chickpeas/garbanzo beans • Edamame • Lentils • Seitan • Tempeh • Tofu	• Amaranth • Barley • Brown rice • Buckwheat • Bulgur • Quinoa • Sorghum • Spelt • Teff • Wild rice	• Cheese (like Feta, parmesan, goat, gorgonzola, or sharp cheddar) • Grilled or baked chicken or fish • Nuts • Olives • Pita Chips • Seeds • Sliced apples or pears • Slivered fennel • Sprinkle of Canadian bacon	• Avocado-based dressing • Dried oregano • Fresh lemon squeeze • Greek yogurt based dressing • Italian seasoning • Olive oil & vinegar (balsamic, red wine, apple cider) • Olive oil & lemon or lime • Pesto • Tahini dressing

Try some of these plant-based recipes, from MelissasHealthyLiving.com and modify them to add grains, protein, or veggies as needed:

- Black beans, tomatoes and artichokes, a 3-minute meal
- Creamy autumn harvest soup
- Easy bean tacos
- Easy salads
- Easy yummy lentil soup
- Ginger honey tofu
- Kale mango and black bean salad
- Lentil, tomato, and feta salad
- Marian's bean salad
- Quick and easy quinoa black bean and corn salsa
- Sweet potato mac-n-cheese
- Tasty pesto garbanzo bean salad
- Yummy chopped quinoa salad
- Zesty quinoa holiday stuffing

Mix-and-Match Smoothies

Mix and match these ingredients to create your own balanced smoothie! Choose fruits and vegetables that are different colors to get a variety of phytochemicals. Opting for a whey protein base will help ensure your smoothie contains high-quality protein. You can also add in a portion of a plant-based protein booster, like pea protein. Smoothies make for a great post-workout snack or meal that is refreshing and packed with nutrients, protein, carbohydrates, and fluids. Want a little more spice in your life and in your smoothie? Look through the list of extra flavor add-ons for some ideas. Sip on your smoothie from a glass or mix it up by swapping your glass for a bowl and spoon.

Tip: When you have seasonal access, find a local farmer's market or farm/produce stand to pick out smoothie ingredients that are in season – they'll be at their peak ripeness and loaded with flavor!

Don't shy away from frozen fruit or veggies when time is tight! They're prewashed, which will save you time, and flash frozen for maximum nutrient content.

Check out these additional recipes on MelissasHealthyLiving.com:

- Apple kale lime smoothie

7.2 - Mix-and-Match Smoothies				
Step 1: Choose your fruit	**Step 2:** Choose your veggies	**Step 3:** Choose a base	**Step 4:** Add in a plant-based protein boost	**Step 5:** Optional flavor add-ons
• Apple • Banana • Berries (strawberry, blueberry, blackberry, raspberry) • Cherries • Dried dates • Grapefruit • Pear • Grapes • Kiwi • Mango • Nectarine • Orange • Peach • Persimmon • Pineapple • Pomegranate seeds • Watermelon	• Avocado • Beet • Bell pepper • Carrot • Cauliflower • Celery • Cucumber • Leafy greens (spinach, kale, arugula) • Peas • Pumpkin puree • Roasted sweet potato	• Coconut water • Greek yogurt (nonfat or low-fat) • Milk (nonfat or low-fat) • Milk alternatives (almond, rice, soy, hemp, etc.) • Water	• Chia seeds • Flax meal • Pea protein • Hemp seeds • Nut butter • Oatmeal, oats • Pre-formulated plant protein powders* • Pumpkin seed butter • Pumpkin seeds • Spirulina powder • Sunflower butter • Walnuts	• Cacao nibs • Clove • Allspice • Cocoa powder • Fresh lemon or lime juice • Fresh mint leaves • Fresh parsley • Ginger root (powdered or fresh) • Granola • Honey • Nutmeg • Shredded coconut • Turmeric (powdered or fresh) • Vanilla extract

*Check the ingredient label on any pre-formulated plant protein powders and keep your eye out for excess added sugar or artificial sweeteners.

- Ginger turmeric lime smoothie
- Pineapple parsley green smoothie
- Pumpkin smoothie
- Purple power smoothie
- Refreshing green smoothie

Check out the companion recipe book for over 100 tasty recipes and their nutrition values.

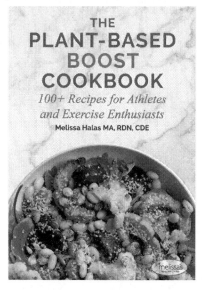

THE
PLANT-BASED BOOST COOKBOOK
100+ Recipes for Athletes and Exercise Enthusiasts
Melissa Halas MA, RDN, CDE

melissas

References

1.   US Department of Health and Human Services. Physical Activity Guidelines for Americans. US Department of Health and Human Services website. https://www. hhs.gov/fitness/be-active/physical-activity-guidelines-for-americans/index.html. Accessed March 1, 2019.

2.   Kreher JB, Schwartz JB. Overtraining syndrome: a practical guide. *Sports Health*. 2012;4(2):128-138. doi:10.1177/1941738111434406

3.   Ferrari HG, Gobatto CA, Manchado-Gobatto FB. Training load, immune system, upper respiratory symptoms and performance in well-trained cyclists throughout a competitive season. *Biol Sport*. 2013;30(4):289-294. doi:10.5604/20831862.1077555

4.   Minihane AM, Vinoy S, Russell WR, et al. Low-grade inflammation, diet composition and health: current research evidence and its translation. *Br J Nutr*. 2015;114(7):999-1012. doi:10.1017/S0007114515002093

5.   Romagnolo DF, Selmin OI. Mediterranean Diet and Prevention of Chronic Diseases. *Nutr Today*. 2017;52(5):208-222. doi:10.1097/NT.0000000000000228

6.   Dinu M, Abbate R, Gensini GF, Casini A, Sofi F. Vegetarian, vegan diets and multiple health outcomes: A systematic review with meta-analysis of observational studies. *Crit Rev Food Sci Nutr*. 2017;57(17):3640-3649. doi:10.1080/10408398.2016.113 8447

7.   Kanter M. High-Quality Carbohydrates and Physical Performance: Expert Panel Report. *Nutr Today*. 2018;53(1):35-39. doi:10.1097/NT.0000000000000238

8.   Hawley JA, Leckey JJ. Carbohydrate Dependence During Prolonged, Intense Endurance Exercise. *Sport Med*. 2015;45(S1):5-12. doi:10.1007/s40279-015-0400-1

9.   Barnard N, Goldman D, Loomis J, et al. Plant-Based Diets for Cardiovascular Safety and Performance in Endurance Sports. *Nutrients*. 2019;11(1):130. doi:10.3390/ nu11010130

10.   Craddock JC, Probst YC, Peoples GE. Vegetarian and Omnivorous Nutrition— Comparing Physical Performance. *Int J Sport Nutr Exerc Metab*. 2016;26(3):212-220. doi:10.1123/ijsnem.2015-0231

11.   Venderley AM, Campbell WW. Vegetarian Diets: nutritional considerations for athletes. *Sport Med*. 2006;36(4):293-305. doi:10.2165/00007256-200636040-00002

12.   Wise J, Vennard D. It's All in a Name: How to Boost the Sales of Plant-Based Menu Items. World Resources Institute website. https://www.wri.org/news/its-all-name-how-boost-sales-plant-based-menu-items.

13.   Lynch H, Johnston C, Wharton C, Lynch H, Johnston C, Wharton C. Plant-Based Diets: Considerations for Environmental Impact, Protein Quality, and Exercise Performance. *Nutrients*. 2018;10(12):1841. doi:10.3390/nu10121841

14.   Food and Agricultural Organization of the United Nations. Key facts and findings. Food and Agricultural Organization of the United Nations website. http://www.fao.org/news/story/en/item/197623/icode/. Accessed March 15, 2019.

15.   Jay J. Easiest climate-friendly comfort food: Black Beans and Rice - Meals 4 The Planet. Meals for the Planet website. https://meals4planet.org/recipe/easiest-climate-friendly-comfort-food-black-beans-and-rice/. Accessed March 15, 2019.

16.   Ranganathan J, Waite R, Searchinger T, Hanson C. How to Sustainably Feed 10 Billion People by 2050, in 21 Charts. World Resources Institute website. https://www.wri.org/blog/2018/12/how-sustainably-feed-10-billion-people-2050-21-charts. Accessed March 15, 2019.

17.   Heller MC, Keoleian GA. Greenhouse Gas Emission Estimates of U.S. Dietary Choices and Food Loss. *J Ind Ecol*. 2015;19(3):391-401. doi:10.1111/jiec.12174

18.   Rosenbloom CA, Coleman EJ, Academy of Nutrition and Dietetics. *Sports Nutrition: A Practice Manual for Professionals. 5th ed.* Chicago, IL: Academy of Nutrition and Dietetics; 2012.

19.   Dutchen S. What Do Fats Do in the Body? - Inside Life Science Series. National Institute of General Medical Sciences website. https://www.nigms.nih.gov/education/Inside-Life-Science/Pages/what-do-fats-do-in-the-body.aspx.   Published 2010. Accessed October 2, 2018.

20.   Gropper SS, Smith JL. *Advanced Nutrition and Human Metabolism*. 6th ed. Belmont, CA: Wadsworth/Cengage Learning; 2013.

21.   Dai Z, Niu J, Zhang Y, Jacques P, Felson DT. Dietary intake of fibre and risk of knee osteoarthritis in two US prospective cohorts. *Ann Rheum Dis*. 2017;76(8):1411-1419. doi:10.1136/annrheumdis-2016-210810

22.   Clinton CM, O'Brien S, Law J, Renier CM, Wendt MR. Whole-foods, plant-based diet alleviates the symptoms of osteoarthritis. *Arthritis*. 2015;2015:708152. doi:10.1155/2015/708152

23.   United States Department of Agriculture. Nutrients and health benefits. Choose MyPlate website. https://www.choosemyplate.gov/vegetables-nutrients-health. Accessed March 1, 2019.

24. What are Pulses. Pulses website. https://pulses.org/nap/what-are-pulses/. Accessed March 1, 2019.

25. Yadav BS, Sharma A, Yadav RB. Resistant starch content of conventionally boiled and pressure-cooked cereals, legumes and tubers. *J Food Sci Technol*. 2010;47(1):84-88. doi:10.1007/s13197-010-0020-6

26. Birt DF, Boylston T, Hendrich S, et al. Resistant starch: promise for improving human health. *Adv Nutr*. 2013;4(6):587-601. doi:10.3945/an.113.004325

27. American Institute for Cancer Research. AICR's Foods that Fight Cancer - Dry Beans and Peas (Legumes). American Institute for Cancer Research website. http://www.aicr.org/foods-that-fight-cancer/legumes.html. Accessed March 1, 2019.

28. Imran M, Ahmad N, Anjum FM, et al. Potential protective properties of flax lignan secoisolariciresinol diglucoside. *Nutr J*. 2015;14:71. doi:10.1186/s12937-015-0059-3

29. Marrelli M, Conforti F, Araniti F, Statti G. Effects of Saponins on Lipid Metabolism: A Review of Potential Health Benefits in the Treatment of Obesity. *Molecules*. 2016;21(10):1404. doi:10.3390/molecules21101404

30. American Institute for Cancer Research. AICR's Foods that Fight Cancer - Soy. American Institute for Cancer Research website. http://www.aicr.org/foods-that-fight-cancer/soy.html. Accessed April 4, 2019.

31. Nechuta SJ, Caan BJ, Chen WY, et al. Soy food intake after diagnosis of breast cancer and survival: an in-depth analysis of combined evidence from cohort studies of US and Chinese women. *Am J Clin Nutr*. 2012;96(1):123-132. doi:10.3945/ajcn.112.035972

32. van Die MD, Bone KM, Williams SG, Pirotta M V. Soy and soy isoflavones in prostate cancer: a systematic review and meta-analysis of randomized controlled trials. *BJU Int*. 2014;113(5b):E119-E130. doi:10.1111/bju.12435

33. American Institute for Cancer Research. AICR's Foods that Fight Cancer. American Institute for Cancer Research website. http://www.aicr.org/foods-that-fight-cancer/. Published 2016. Accessed March 1, 2019.

34. Guha N, Kwan ML, Quesenberry CP, Weltzien EK, Castillo AL, Caan BJ. Soy isoflavones and risk of cancer recurrence in a cohort of breast cancer survivors: the Life After Cancer Epidemiology study. *Breast Cancer Res Treat*. 2009;118(2):395-405. doi:10.1007/s10549-009-0321-5

35. Sathyapalan T, Manuchehri AM, Thatcher NJ, et al. The Effect of Soy Phytoestrogen Supplementation on Thyroid Status and Cardiovascular Risk Markers in Patients with Subclinical Hypothyroidism: A Randomized, Double-Blind, Crossover Study. *J Clin Endocrinol Metab*. 2011;96(5):1442-1449. doi:10.1210/jc.2010-2255

36.   Messina M, Redmond G. Effects of Soy Protein and Soybean Isoflavones on Thyroid Function in Healthy Adults and Hypothyroid Patients: A Review of the Relevant Literature. *Thyroid*. 2006;16(3):249-258. doi:10.1089/thy.2006.16.249

37.   National Institutes of Health Office of Dietary Supplements. Calcium Fact Sheet for Health Professionals. National Institutes of Health Office of Dietary Supplements website. https://ods.od.nih.gov/factsheets/Calcium-HealthProfessional/. Accessed December 11, 2018.

38.   Johnson G. *New Soybean Oil Health Claim Based on Solid Body of Evidence. Soy Connection website.* 2018. https://www.soyconnection.com/healthprofessionals/ newsletter/health-nutrition-newsletter/newsletter-article-list/health-nutrition- -winter-2018/2018/08/02/new-soybean-oil-health-claim-based-on-solid-body- of-evidence. Accessed March 2, 2019.

39.   Eggcyclopedia - Biological Value. Incredible Egg website. https://www.incredibleegg.org/eggcyclopedia/b/biological-value/. Accessed October 2, 2018.

40.   Pulse Canada. *Protein Quality of Cooked Pulses*. Pulse Canada website. http:// www.pulsecanada.com/wp-content/uploads/2017/09/Pulses-and-Protein-Quality. pdf. Accessed March 1, 2019.

41.   Webb D. Athletes and Protein Intake. Today's Dietitian website. https://www. todaysdietitian.com/newarchives/060114p22.shtml. Published 2014.

42.   Lee WT, Weisell R, Albert J, Tomé D, Kurpad A V, Uauy R. Research Approaches and Methods for Evaluating the Protein Quality of Human Foods Proposed by an FAO Expert Working Group in 2014. *J Nutr*. 2016;146(5):929-932. doi:10.3945/jn.115.222109

43.   Protein %DV - PER & PDCAAS. ESHA Research website. https://esha.zendesk. com/hc/en-us/articles/202915018-Protein-DV-PER-PDCAAS. Accessed October 2, 2018.

44.   Mathai JK, Liu Y, Stein HH. Values for digestible indispensable amino acid scores (DIAAS) for some dairy and plant proteins may better describe protein quality than values calculated using the concept for protein digestibility-corrected amino acid scores (PDCAAS). *Br J Nutr*. 2017;117(04):490-499. doi:10.1017/S0007114517000125

45.   FAO Expert Consultation. Dietary protein quality evaluation in human nutrition. FAO Food and Nutrition Paper 92. http://www.fao.org/ag/humannutrition/35978- 02317b979a686a57aa4593304ffc17f06.pdf. Accessed March 1, 2019.

46.   The power of high-quality protein. Chobani Foodservice website. https://chobanifoodservice.com/whats-trending/the-power-of-high-quality-protein. Accessed March 1, 2019.

47.   National Research Council (US) Subcommittee on the Tenth Edition of the Recommended Dietary Allowances. Recommended Dietary Allowances: 10th ed. Washington (DC): National Academies Press (US); 1989.

48.   Phillips SM. Current Concepts and Unresolved Questions in Dietary Protein Requirements and Supplements in Adults. *Front Nutr.* 2017;4:13. doi:10.3389/fnut.2017.00013

49.   European Dairy Association (EDA). *Dairy: A Source of High Quality Protein.* European Dairy Association website. http://eda.euromilk.org/old-pages/read/article/dairy-a-source-of-high-quality-protein.html. Accessed March 1, 2019.

50.   Cahill WM, Schroeder LJ, Smith AH. Digestibility and biological value of soybean protein in whole soybeans, soybean floor, and soybean milk. *J Nutr.* 1944;28:209-218. doi: 19441403376

51.   Marinangeli CPF, House JD. Potential impact of the digestible indispensable amino acid score as a measure of protein quality on dietary regulations and health. *Nutr Rev.* 2017;75(8):658-667. doi:10.1093/nutrit/nux025

52.   Murlin JR, Cowgill GR, Wistar Institute of Anatomy and Biology. *The Journal of Nutrition.* 1944;28.

53.   Ghassem M. Protein quality of selected edible animal and plant protein sources using rat bio-assay. *Int Food Res J.* 2010;17:303-308.

54.   Rizzo G, Baroni L. Soy, Soy Foods and Their Role in Vegetarian Diets. *Nutrients.* 2018;10(1):43. doi:10.3390/nu10010043

55.   Hughes GJ, Ryan DJ, Mukherjea R, Schasteen CS. Protein Digestibility-Corrected Amino Acid Scores (PDCAAS) for Soy Protein Isolates and Concentrate: Criteria for Evaluation. *J Agric Food Chem.* 2011;59(23):12707-12712. doi:10.1021/jf203220v

56.   WHO/FAO/UNU Expert Consultation. *WHO Technical Report Series 935 Protein and Amino Acid Requirements in Human Nutrition, Report of a Joint WHO/FAO/UNU Expert Consultation.* 2007. Accessed March 1, 2019.

57.   Jäger R, Kerksick CM, Campbell BI, et al. International Society of Sports Nutrition Position Stand: protein and exercise. *J Int Soc Sports Nutr.* 2017;14(1):20. doi:10.1186/s12970-017-0177-8

58.   Academy of Nutrition and Dietetics. Safety and Effectiveness of Selected Dietary Supplements and Ergogenic Aids - Nutrition Care Manual. Sports Nutrition Care Manual website. https://www.nutritioncaremanual.org/topic.cfm?ncm_toc_id=273812. Accessed March 1, 2019.

59.   Maughan RJ, IOC Medical Commission. *Sports Nutrition.* Wiley-Blackwell; 2014.

60.   Sports Dietitians Australia. Fact Sheet - *Protein and Amino Acid Supplementation*. https://www.sportsdietitians.com.au/wp-content/uploads/2015/04/110701-Protein-Supplementation_General.pdf. 2011. Accessed October 2, 2018.

61.   Breen L, Phillips SM. Skeletal muscle protein metabolism in the elderly: Interventions to counteract the "anabolic resistance" of ageing. *Nutr Metab (Lond)*. 2011;8:68. doi:10.1186/1743-7075-8-68

62.   United States Department of Agriculture Agricultural Research Service. USDA Food Composition Databases. USDA Food Composition Databases website. https://ndb.nal.usda.gov/ndb/. Accessed March 1, 2019.

63.   van Vliet S, Burd NA, van Loon LJ. The Skeletal Muscle Anabolic Response to Plant- versus Animal-Based Protein Consumption. *J Nutr*. 2015;145(9):1981-1991. doi:10.3945/jn.114.204305

64.   Egan B. Protein intake for athletes and active adults: Current concepts and controversies. *Nutr Bull*. 2016;41(3):202-213. doi:10.1111/nbu.12215

65.   United States Department of Agriculture Agricultural Research Service. Food Composition Databases Show Foods List. USDA Food Composition Databases website. https://ndb.nal.usda.gov/ndb/search/list. Accessed October 2, 2018.

66.   Ullah R, Nadeem M, Khalique A, et al. Nutritional and therapeutic perspectives of Chia (Salvia hispanica L.): a review. *J Food Sci Technol*. 2016;53(4):1750-1758. doi:10.1007/s13197-015-1967-0

67.   Zaraska M. Raising the Steaks: How One City in the Netherlands Wants to Feed the World. Discover Magazine. http://discovermagazine.com/2019/apr/raising-the-steaks. Published 2019. Accessed April 4, 2019.

68.   de Beukelaar MFA, Zeinstra GG, Mes JJ, Fischer ARH. Duckweed as human food. The influence of meal context and information on duckweed acceptability of Dutch consumers. *Food Qual Prefer*. 2019;71:76-86. doi:10.1016/J.FOODQUAL.2018.06.005

69.   Tarver T. Palatable Proteins for Complex Palates. *Inst Food Technol*. 2016;70(3). http://www.ift.org/Food-Technology/Past-Issues/2016/March/Features/palatable-proteins-for-complex-palates.aspx. Accessed April 4, 2019.

70.   Owen N, Sparling PB, Healy GN, Dunstan DW, Matthews CE. Sedentary behavior: emerging evidence for a new health risk. *Mayo Clin Proc*. 2010;85(12):1138-1141. doi:10.4065/mcp.2010.0444

71.   Jetté M, Sidney K, Blümchen G. Metabolic equivalents (METS) in exercise testing, exercise prescription, and evaluation of functional capacity. *Clin Cardiol*. 1990;13(8):555-565. doi: 10.1002/clc.4960130809

72. Center for Disease Control and Prevention. *General Physical Activities Defined by Level of Intensity.* https://www.cdc.gov/nccdphp/dnpa/physical/pdf/pa_intensity_table_2_1.pdf. Accessed March 1, 2019.

73. Institute of Medicine. *Dietary Reference Intakes: The Essential Guide to Nutrient Requirements Dietary Reference Intakes DRI.* Washington, DC: The National Academies Press; 2006. http://www.nap.edu/catalog/11537.html. Accessed October 2, 2018.

74. Helms ER, Aragon AA, Fitschen PJ. Evidence-based recommendations for natural bodybuilding contest preparation: nutrition and supplementation. *J Int Soc Sports Nutr.* 2014;11:20. doi:10.1186/1550-2783-11-20

75. Helms ER, Zinn C, Rowlands DS, Brown SR. A Systematic Review of Dietary Protein during Caloric Restriction in Resistance Trained Lean Athletes: A Case for Higher Intakes. *Int J Sport Nutr Exerc Metab.* 2014;24(2):127-138. doi:10.1123/ijsnem.2013-0054

76. Rodriguez NR. Introduction to Protein Summit 2.0: continued exploration of the impact of high-quality protein on optimal health. *Am J Clin Nutr.* 2015;101(6):1317S-1319S. doi:10.3945/ajcn.114.083980

77. Coleman E. *Eating for Endurance. 4th ed.* Bull Pub. Co; 2003.

78. Thomas DT, Erdman KA, Burke LM. Nutrition and Athletic Performance. *Med Sci Sport Exerc.* 2016;48(3):543-568. doi:10.1249/MSS.0000000000000852

79. Kerksick CM, Wilborn CD, Roberts MD, et al. ISSN exercise & sports nutrition review update: research & recommendations. *J Int Soc Sports Nutr.* 2018;15(1):38. doi:10.1186/s12970-018-0242-y

80. Karpinski C, Rosenbloom C. *Sports Nutrition A Handbook for Professionals.* 6th ed. Chicago, IL: Academy of Nutrition and Dietetics; 2017.

81. Burke L, Deakin V, Allanson B. *Clinical Sports Nutrition.* McGraw Hill. https://trove.nla.gov.au/work/4017911.

82. Helms ER, Aragon AA, Fitschen PJ. Evidence-based recommendations for natural bodybuilding contest preparation: nutrition and supplementation. *J Int Soc Sports Nutr.* 2014;11(1):20. doi:10.1186/1550-2783-11-20

83. Schoenfeld BJ, Aragon AA. How much protein can the body use in a single meal for muscle-building? Implications for daily protein distribution. *J Int Soc Sports Nutr.* 2018;15(1):10. doi:10.1186/s12970-018-0215-1

84. Williams M, Kreider R, Branch D. *Nutrition for Health, Fitness, & Sport.* New York, NY: McGraw-Hill Education; 2017.

85. U.S. National Library of Medicine. Water in diet: MedlinePlus Medical Encyclopedia. Medline Plus website. https://medlineplus.gov/ency/article/002471.htm. Accessed March 1, 2019.

86. Cheuvront SM, Sawka MN. SSE #97 Hydration Assessment of Athletes. Gatorade Sports Science Institute website. https://www.gssiweb.org/sports-science-exchange/article/sse-97-hydration-assessment-of-athletes. Accessed March 1, 2019.

87. USOC Sport Nutrition Team. Hydration Factsheet. https://www.teamusa.org/nutrition.

88. Sawka MN, Burke LM, Eichner ER, Maughan RJ, Montain SJ, Stachenfeld NS. Exercise and Fluid Replacement. *Med Sci Sport Exerc*. 2007;39(2):377-390. doi:10.1249/mss.0b013e31802ca597

89. Maughan RJ, Burke LM, Dvorak J, et al. IOC consensus statement: dietary supplements and the high-performance athlete. *Br J Sports Med*. 2018;52(7):439-455. doi:10.1136/bjsports-2018-099027

90. Skratch Labs Sport Hydration Drink Mix. Skratch Labs website. https://www.skratchlabs.com/collections/drinks/products/sport-hydration-drink-mix?variant=42591626629. Accessed March 3, 2019.

91. World Health Organization. WHO calls on countries to reduce sugars intake among adults and children. *WHO website*. 2016. https://www.who.int/mediacentre/news/releases/2015/sugar-guideline/en/. Accessed March 1, 2019.

92. Schnabel L, Kesse-Guyot E, Allès B, et al. Association Between Ultraprocessed Food Consumption and Risk of Mortality Among Middle-aged Adults in France. *JAMA Intern Med*. February 2019. doi:10.1001/jamainternmed.2018.7289

93. National Institutes of Health Office of Dietary Supplements. Magnesium Fact Sheet for Health Professionals. National Institutes of Health Office of Dietary Supplements website. https://ods.od.nih.gov/factsheets/Magnesium-HealthProfessional/. Accessed December 11, 2018.

94. National Institutes of Health Office of Dietary Supplements (ODS). https://ods.od.nih.gov/. Accessed March 1, 2019.

95. US Food and Drug Administration. CFR - Code of Federal Regulations Title 21. US Food and Drug Administration website. https://www.accessdata.fda.gov/scripts/cdrh/cfdocs/cfcfr/cfrsearch.cfm?fr=101.54. Accessed March 1, 2019.

96. The Whole Grains Council. Barley – February Grain of the Month. The Whole Grains Council website. https://wholegrainscouncil.org/whole-grains-101/grain-month-calendar/barley---february-grain-month. Accessed March 1, 2019.

97.   The Whole Grains Council. Buckwheat - December Grain of the Month. The Whole Grains Council website. https://wholegrainscouncil.org/whole-grains-101/grain-month-calendar/buckwheat-december-grain-month. Accessed March 1, 2019.

98.   Webster A. Gut Check: Prebiotics and the Microbiome. International Food Information Council Foundation website. https://foodinsight.org/gut-check-prebiotics-and-the-microbiome/. Accessed April 4, 2019.

99.   Giménez-Bastida JA, Zieliński H. Buckwheat as a Functional Food and Its Effects on Health. *J Agric Food Chem*. 2015;63(36):7896-7913. doi:10.1021/acs.jafc.5b02498

100. Cooper R. Re-discovering ancient wheat varieties as functional foods. *J Tradit Complement Med*. 2015;5(3):138-143. doi:10.1016/j.jtcme.2015.02.004

101. The Trademark. KAMUT® Khorasan Wheat website. https://www.kamut.com/en/discover/the-trademark. Accessed March 1, 2019.

102. Tangney CC, Rasmussen HE. Polyphenols, inflammation, and cardiovascular disease. *Curr Atheroscler Rep*. 2013;15(5):324. doi:10.1007/s11883-013-0324-x

103. Case S. Are Oats OK on the Gluten-Free Diet? Allergic Living website. https://www.allergicliving.com/2010/07/02/ask-the-celiac-expert-are-oats-ok/. Published 2010. Accessed March 1, 2019.

104. Center for Food Safety and Applied Nutrition US Food & Drug Administration. FDA Statement on Testing and Analysis of Arsenic in Rice and Rice Products. US Food & Drug Administration website. https://www.fda.gov/food/metals/fda-statement-testing-and-analysis-arsenic-rice-and-rice-products. Accessed March 1, 2019.

105. Marcason W. What Are the Current Findings Concerning Arsenic in Foods? *J Acad Nutr Diet*. 2015;115:1028. doi:10.1016/j.jand.2015.04.011

106. *Food Safety and Sustainability Center. Report: Analysis of Arsenic in Rice and Other Grains*. 2014. http://greenerchoices.org/wp-content/uploads/2016/08/CR_FSASC_Arsenic_Analysis_Nov2014.pdf. Accessed March 1, 2019.

107. Consumer Reports. How Much Arsenic Is in Your Rice? https://www.consumer-reports.org/cro/magazine/2015/01/how-much-arsenic-is-in-your-rice/index.htm. Published 2014. Accessed March 1, 2019.

108. The Whole Grains Council. Rye + Triticale August Grains of the Month. The Whole Grains Council website. https://wholegrainscouncil.org/whole-grains-101/grain-month-calendar/rye-triticale-august-grains-month. Accessed March 1, 2019.

109. Tiwari BK, Brunton NP, Brennan CS, eds. *Handbook of Plant Food Phytochemicals*. Oxford: John Wiley & Sons Ltd; 2013. doi:10.1002/9781118464717

110.   Yilmaz HO, Arslan M. *Teff: Nutritional Compounds and Effects on Human Health.* *Acta Scientific Medical Sciences.* 2018;2.9:15-18.

111.   Baye K. Teff: Nutrient Composition and Health Benefits. https://www.research-gate.net/publication/266316373_Teff_Nutrient_Composition_and_Health_Benefits. Accessed March 15, 2019.

112.   The Whole Grains Council. Definition of a Whole Grain. The Whole Grains Council website. https://wholegrainscouncil.org/definition-whole-grain. Accessed April 4, 2019.

113.   The Whole Grains Council. Whole White Wheat FAQ. The Whole Grains Council website.   https://wholegrainscouncil.org/whole-grains-101/whats-whole-grain-refined-grain/whole-white-wheat-faq. Accessed April 4, 2019.

114.   The Whole Grains Council. Compare Nutrients in Various Grains. The Whole Grains Council website. https://wholegrainscouncil.org/whole-grains-101/health-studies-health-benefits/compare-nutrients-various-grains. Accessed October 2, 2018.

115.   The Whole Grains Council. https://wholegrainscouncil.org/. The Whole Grains Council website. Accessed March 1, 2019.

116.   University Dining Services. Grains Cooking Chart. UC Davis website. https://shcs.ucdavis.edu/one-balanced-kitchen.

117.   The Whole Grains Council. Cooking Whole Grains. The Whole Grains Council website. https://wholegrainscouncil.org/recipes/cooking-whole-grains. Accessed March 15, 2019.

118.   Boeckmann C. How to Cook Grains Chart - How to Cook Barley, Buckwheat, And Other Whole Grains. The Old Farmer's Almanac website. https://www.almanac.com/content/how-to-cook-whole-grains. Accessed March 15, 2019.

119.   Parker K. How to Cook Brown Rice Perfectly. EatingWell website. http://www.eatingwell.com/article/67554/how-to-cook-brown-rice-perfectly/.   Accessed March 15, 2019.

120. Basic Preparation Instructions for Organic Whole Grain Kamut® Berries Recipe. Bob's Red Mill website. https://www.bobsredmill.com/recipes/how-to-make/basic-preparation-instructions-for-organic-kamut-berries/. Accessed March 15, 2019.

121.   Bob's Red Mill Organic Polenta Corn Grits -- 24 oz. Vitacost website. https://www.vitacost.com/bobs-red-mill-organic-polenta-corn-grits. Accessed March 15, 2019.

122.   Basic Preparation Instructions for Gluten Free Sorghum Grain Recipe. Bob's Red Mill website. https://www.bobsredmill.com/recipes/how-to-make/basic-preparation-instructions-for-gluten-free-sorghum-grain/. Accessed March 15, 2019.

123.   Schardt D. Arsenic Found in Almost Every Rice-containing Food. Nutrition Action website. https://www.nutritionaction.com/daily/food-safety/arsenic-found-in-almost-every-rice-containing-food/. Published 2013. Accessed March 1, 2019.

124.   Gan Y, Liang C, Wang X, McConkey B. Lowering carbon footprint of durum wheat by diversifying cropping systems. *F Crop Res*. 2011;122(3):199-206. doi:10.1016/J.FCR.2011.03.020

125.   Li J, Liu K, Zhang J, et al. Soil–Plant Indices Help Explain Legume Response to Crop Rotation in a Semiarid Environment. *Front Plant Sci*. 2018;9:1488. doi:10.3389/fpls.2018.01488

126.   Eat This, Not That! Editors. 9 Best Pastas for Weight Loss. Eat This, Not That! Website. https://www.eatthis.com/9-best-pasta-weight-loss/. Accessed October 2, 2018.

127.   Pow! Pasta Red Lentil Rotini. Ancient Harvest website. https://ancientharvest.com/product/pow-pasta-red-lentil-rotini/. Accessed March 1, 2019.

128.   Ancient Harvest POW! Gluten Free Protein Pasta, Black Bean and Quinoa Elbows, 8 oz (Pack of 6). Amazon website. https://www.amazon.com/Ancient-Harvest-Gluten-Protein-Quinoa/dp/B00VV8EEUW. Accessed March 1, 2019.

129.   Eden Foods Kamut® & Quinoa Twisted Pair®, Organic, 100% Whole Grain. Eden Foods website. https://www.edenfoods.com/store/kamutr-quinoa-twisted-pairr-organic-100-whole-grain.html. Accessed March 1, 2019.

130.   Eden Foods Kamut® Spaghetti, 100% Whole Grain, Organic. Eden Foods website. https://www.edenfoods.com/store/kamutr-spaghetti-100-whole-grain-organic.html. Accessed March 1, 2019.

131.   Eden Foods Kamut® & Buckwheat Rigatoni, Organic, 100% Whole Grain. Eden Foods website. https://www.edenfoods.com/store/kamutr-buckwheat-rigatoni-organic-100-whole-grain.html. Accessed March 1, 2019.

132.   Eden Foods Spelt & Buckwheat Gemelli, Organic, 100% Whole Grain. Eden Foods website. https://www.edenfoods.com/store/spelt-buckwheat-gemelli-organic-100-whole-grain.html. Accessed March 1, 2019.

133.   Whole Grain Flours, Oats & Cereals. Bob's Red Mill website. https://www.bobsredmill.com/. Accessed March 1, 2019.

134. Bowman SA, Clemens JC, Friday JE, Lynch KL, Moshfegh AJ. *Food Patterns Equivalents Database 2013-14: Methodology and User Guide*. 2017. https://www.ars.usda.gov/ARSUserFiles/80400530/pdf/fped/FPED_1314.pdf. Accessed March 15, 2019.

135. Barilla Chickpea Rotini. Barilla website. https://www.barilla.com/en-us/products/pasta/legume/chickpea-rotini. Accessed March 15, 2019.

136. Product Details O Organics Organic Tofu Extra Firm - 14 Oz. Vons website. https://shop.vons.com/product-details.960027626.html. Accessed March 1, 2019.

137. Seafood Counter Fish Salmon Atlantic Fillet Color Added Farmed Fresh Service Counter - 1.50 LB. Safeway website. https://shop.safeway.com/product-details.960267461.html. Accessed March 15, 2019.

138. United States Department of Agriculture Agricultural Research Service. Chicken Turkey Nutrition Facts. USDA Food Composition Databases website. https://www.fsis.usda.gov/shared/PDF/Chicken_Turkey_Nutrition_Facts.pdf. Published 2011. Accessed March 15, 2019.

139. Product Details Foster Farms Fresh & Natural Turkey Breast Tenderloins Boneless & Skinless - 1.25 Lb. Safeway website. https://shop.safeway.com/product-details.960153083.html?r=https%3A%2F%2Falbertsons.okta.com%2Fsso%2Fsaml2%2F00a1h67i2yVn6pj5g2p7. Accessed March 15, 2019.

140. Product Details Jennie-O Turkey Store Turkey Ground Turkey 93% Lean 7% Fat - 16 Oz. Safeway website. https://shop.safeway.com/product-details.960138390.html. Accessed March 15, 2019.

141. Meat Counter Chicken Breast Boneless Skinless Hand Trimmed 1 Count Service Case - 1.50 lb. Safeway website. https://shop.safeway.com/product-details.960262533.html. Accessed March 15, 2019.

142. Foster Farms Ground Chicken Breast - 16oz. Target website. https://www.target.com/p/foster-farms-ground-chicken-breast-16oz/-/A-50023098?ref=tgt_adv_XS000000&AFID=google_pla_df&fndsrc=tgtao&CPNG=PLA_Grocery%2BEssentials%2BShopping_Local&adgroup=SC_Grocery&LID=700000001170770pgs&network=g&device=c&location=9031962. Accessed March 15, 2019.

143. Search Results: ground beef. Safeway website. https://shop.safeway.com/search-results.html?q=ground beef&r=https%3A%2F%2Falbertsons.okta.com%2Fsso%2Fsaml2%2F00a1h67i2yVn6pj5g2p7. Accessed March 15, 2019.

144. Search Results: flank steak. Safeway website. https://shop.safeway.com/search-results.html?q=flank steak. Accessed March 15, 2019.

145. van Buul VJ, Brouns FJPH. Health effects of wheat lectins: A review. *J Cereal Sci*. 2014;59(2):112-117. doi:10.1016/J.JCS.2014.01.010

146. Lajolo FM, Genovese MI. Nutritional significance of lectins and enzyme inhibitors from legumes. *J Agric Food Chem*. 2002;50(22):6592-6598. http://www.ncbi.nlm.nih.gov/pubmed/12381157. Accessed March 1, 2019.

147. Rodhouse JC, Haugh CA, Roberts D, Gilbert RJ. Red kidney bean poisoning in the UK: an analysis of 50 suspected incidents between 1976 and 1989. *Epidemiol Infect*. 1990;105(3):485-491. http://www.ncbi.nlm.nih.gov/pubmed/2249712. Accessed March 1, 2019.

148. Singh RS, Kaur HP, Kanwar JR. Mushroom Lectins as Promising Anticancer Substances. *Curr Protein Pept Sci*. 2016;17(8):797-807. http://www.ncbi.nlm.nih.gov/pubmed/26916164. Accessed March 1, 2019.

149. Shi L, Arntfield SD, Nickerson M. Changes in levels of phytic acid, lectins and oxalates during soaking and cooking of Canadian pulses. *Food Res Int*. 2018;107:660-668. doi:10.1016/J.FOODRES.2018.02.056

150. Amidor T. Ask the Expert: Clearing Up Lectin Misconceptions. Today's Dietitian Magazine website. https://www.todaysdietitian.com/newarchives/1017p10.shtml#at_pco=smlwn-1.0&at_si=5c5b3441fae42ce2&at_ab=per-2&at_pos=0&at_tot=1. Published 2017. Accessed March 1, 2019.

151. Mahan LK, Escott-Stump S, Raymond JL, Krause M V. *Krause's Food and the Nutrition Care Process*. Elsevier/Saunders; 2012.

152. *U.S. Food and Drug Administration. Nutrition Facts Label, Dietary Fiber*. 2018. https://www.accessdata.fda.gov/scripts/interactivenutritionfactslabel/factsheets/Dietary_Fiber.pdf. Accessed March 15, 2019.

153. U.S. Department of Health and Human Services and U.S. Department of Agriculture. 2015–2020 Dietary Guidelines for Americans. 8th ed. December 2015. https://health.gov/dietaryguidelines/2015/guidelines/. Accessed October 2, 2018.

154. de Oliveira EP, Burini RC, Jeukendrup A. Gastrointestinal Complaints During Exercise: Prevalence, Etiology, and Nutritional Recommendations. *Sport Med*. 2014;44(S1):79-85. doi:10.1007/s40279-014-0153-2

155. Jeukendrup A. New position statement on Nutrition and Athletic Performance. Mysportscience website. http://www.mysportscience.com/single-post/2016/04/02/New-position-statement-on-Nutrition-and-Athletic-Performance. Published 2016. Accessed October 2, 2018.

156. World Health Organization. What is Moderate-intensity and Vigorous-intensity Physical Activity? *World Health Organization website*. 2014. https://www.who.int/dietphysicalactivity/physical_activity_intensity/en/. Accessed March 1, 2019.

157. Murray B, Rosenbloom C. Fundamentals of glycogen metabolism for coaches and athletes. *Nutr Rev*. 2018;76(4):243-259. doi:10.1093/nutrit/nuy001

158. Tardie G. Glycogen Replenishment After Exhaustive Exercise. *Sport J.* 1998;20. http://thesportjournal.org/article/glycogen-replenishment-after-exhaustive-exercise/. Accessed March 1, 2019.

159. Kerksick C, Harvey T, Stout J, et al. International Society of Sports Nutrition position stand: Nutrient timing. *J Int Soc Sports Nutr.* 2008;5(1):17. doi:10.1186/1550-2783-5-17

160. Burke LM, Hawley JA, S Wong SH, Jeukendrup AE. Carbohydrates for training and competition. *J Sports Sci.* 2011;29:17-27. doi:10.1080/02640414.2011.585473

161. Jeukendrup A. Carb loading: what is new? Mysportscience website. http://www.mysportscience.com/single-post/2016/05/12/Carb-loading-what-is-new. Published 2016. Accessed March 1, 2019.

162. McArdle WD, Katch FI, Katch VL. *Sports and exercise nutrition.* Philadelphia, PA. Wolters Kluwer Health/Lippincott Williams & Wilkins. https://trove.nla.gov.au/work/8508241. Accessed October 2, 2018.

163. Burke LM, Jeukendrup AE, Jones AM, Mooses M. Contemporary Nutrition Strategies to Optimize Performance in Distance Runners and Race Walkers. *Int J Sport Nutr Exerc Metab.* February 2019:1-42. doi:10.1123/ijsnem.2019-0004

164. Scarlata K. Low And High Fodmap Diet Checklists. Kate Scarlata website. https://www.katescarlata.com/lowfodmapdietchecklists. Accessed March 15, 2019.

165. Dietitians of Canada, Academy of Nutrition and Dietetics, American College of Sports Medicine. Nutrition and Athletic Performance. https://www.dietitians.ca/Downloads/Public/noap-position-paper.aspx. Accessed October 2, 2018.

166. Canadian Academy of Sports Nutrition. Carbohydrate Loading. Canadian Academy of Sports Nutrition website. https://www.caasn.com/sports-nutrition/sport-nutrition/carbohydrate-loading.html. Accessed October 2, 2018.

167. Caspero A. Protein and the Athlete - How Much Do You Need? Eat Right Academy of Nutrition and Dietetics website. https://www.eatright.org/fitness/sports-and-performance/fueling-your-workout/protein-and-the-athlete. Published 2017. Accessed October 2, 2018.

168. United States Department of Agriculture Agricultural Research Service. Full Report (All Nutrients): UNSWEETENED PEA PROTEIN POWDER, UPC: 039978003607. USDA Food Composition Databases website. https://ndb.nal.usda.gov/ndb/foods/show/45357039?fgcd=&manu=&format=&count=&max=25&offset=&sort=default&order=asc&qlookup=pea+protein&ds=&qt=&qp=&qa=&qn=&q=&ing=. Accessed March 15, 2019.

169. United States Department of Agriculture Agricultural Research Service. Basic Report: 16163, MORI-NU, Tofu, silken, extra firm. USDA Food Composition Databases website. https://ndb.nal.usda.gov/ndb/foods/show/16163?man=&lfacet=&count=&max=25&qlookup=tofu&offset=&sort=default&format=Abridged&reportfmt=other&rptfrm=&ndbno=&nutrient1=&nutrient2=&nutrient3=&subset=&totCount=&measureby=&Qv=2.2&Q331125=1&Qv=1&Q331125=1. Accessed March 15, 2019.

170. Rasane P, Jha A, Sabikhi L, Kumar A, Unnikrishnan VS. Nutritional advantages of oats and opportunities for its processing as value added foods - a review. *J Food Sci Technol*. 2015;52(2):662-675. doi:10.1007/s13197-013-1072-1

171. The Whole Grains Council. Oats – January Grain of the Month. The Whole Grains Council website. https://wholegrainscouncil.org/whole-grains-101/easy-ways-enjoy-whole-grains/grain-month-calendar/oats---january-grain-month. Accessed March 1, 2019.

172. Rogerson D. Vegan diets: practical advice for athletes and exercisers. *J Int Soc Sports Nutr*. 2017;14(1):36. doi:10.1186/s12970-017-0192-9

173. Wang DD, Li Y, Chiuve SE, et al. Association of Specific Dietary Fats With Total and Cause-Specific Mortality. *JAMA Intern Med*. 2016;176(8):1134. doi:10.1001/jamainternmed.2016.2417

174. Oswal A, Yeo G. Leptin and the Control of Body Weight: A Review of Its Diverse Central Targets, Signaling Mechanisms, and Role in the Pathogenesis of Obesity. *Obesity*. 2010;18(2):221-229. doi:10.1038/oby.2009.228

175. Davis A. You Are What You Eat. *The Chemistry of Health*. National Institute of General Medical Sciences website. https://publications.nigms.nih.gov/chemhealth/eat.htm. Accessed October 2, 2018.

176. Bytomski JR. Fueling for Performance. *Sport Heal A Multidiscip Approach*. 2018;10(1):47-53. doi:10.1177/1941738117743913

177. American Heart Association. Monounsaturated Fat. American Heart Association website. https://www.heart.org/en/healthy-living/healthy-eating/eat-smart/fats/monounsaturated-fats. Accessed March 2, 2019.

178. National Institutes of Health Office of Dietary Supplements. Vitamin E Fact Sheet for Health Professionals. National Institutes of Health Office of Dietary Supplements website. https://ods.od.nih.gov/factsheets/VitaminE-HealthProfessional/. Accessed March 1, 2019.

179. American Heart Association. Polyunsaturated Fat. American Heart Association website. https://www.heart.org/en/healthy-living/healthy-eating/eat-smart/fats/polyunsaturated-fats. Accessed March 2, 2019.

180. Franz M. Nutrition, Inflammation, and Disease. Today's Dietitian website. https://www.todaysdietitian.com/newarchives/020314p44.shtml. Accessed March 1, 2019.

181. Jouris KB, McDaniel JL, Weiss EP. The Effect of Omega-3 Fatty Acid Supplementation on the Inflammatory Response to eccentric strength exercise. *J Sports Sci Med.* 2011;10(3):432-438. http://www.ncbi.nlm.nih.gov/pubmed/24150614. Accessed March 15, 2019.

182. Ochi E, Tsuchiya Y, Yanagimoto K. Effect of eicosapentaenoic acids-rich fish oil supplementation on motor nerve function after eccentric contractions. *J Int Soc Sports Nutr.* 2017;14(1):23. doi:10.1186/s12970-017-0176-9

183. Tsuchiya Y, Yanagimoto K, Nakazato K, Hayamizu K, Ochi E. Eicosapentaenoic and docosahexaenoic acids-rich fish oil supplementation attenuates strength loss and limited joint range of motion after eccentric contractions: a randomized, double-blind, placebo-controlled, parallel-group trial. *Eur J Appl Physiol.* 2016;116(6):1179-1188. doi:10.1007/s00421-016-3373-3

184. Corder KE, Newsham KR, McDaniel JL, Ezekiel UR, Weiss EP. Effects of Short-Term Docosahexaenoic Acid Supplementation on Markers of Inflammation after Eccentric Strength Exercise in Women. *J Sports Sci Med.* 2016;15(1):176-183. http://www.ncbi.nlm.nih.gov/pubmed/26957941. Accessed March 15, 2019.

185. Vannice G, Rasmussen H. Position of the Academy of Nutrition and Dietetics: Dietary Fatty Acids for Healthy Adults. *J Acad Nutr Diet.* 2014;114(1):136-153. doi:10.1016/j.jand.2013.11.001

186. National Institutes of Health Office of Dietary Supplements. Omega-3 Fatty Acids Fact Sheet for Professionals. National Institutes of Health Office of Dietary Supplements website. https://ods.od.nih.gov/factsheets/Omega3FattyAcids-HealthProfessional/. Accessed October 2, 2018.

187. SalaVila A, GuaschFerré M, Hu FB, et al. Dietary Linolenic Acid, Marine 3 Fatty Acids, and Mortality in a Population With High Fish Consumption: Findings From the PREvención con DIeta MEDiterránea (PREDIMED) Study. *J Am Heart Assoc.* 2016;5(1). doi:10.1161/JAHA.115.002543

188. National Institutes of Health Office of Dietary Supplements. Omega-3 Fatty Acids Fact Sheet for Consumers. National Institutes of Health Office of Dietary Supplements website. https://ods.od.nih.gov/factsheets/Omega3FattyAcids-Consumer/. Accessed March 1, 2019.

189. World Health Organization. 5. Population nutrient intake goals for preventing diet-related chronic diseases. World Health Organization website. 2007. https://www.who.int/nutrition/topics/5_population_nutrient/en/index13.html. Accessed March 15, 2019.

190. Types of Fat Unsaturated fats. Harvard T.H. Chan School of Public Health website. https://www.hsph.harvard.edu/nutritionsource/what-should-you-eat/fats-and-cholesterol/types-of-fat/. Accessed October 2, 2018.

191. American Heart Association. Saturated Fat. American Heart Association website. http://www.heart.org/en/healthy-living/healthy-eating/eat-smart/fats/saturated-fats. Accessed October 2, 2018.

192. Dietitians Association of Australia. Where do I find saturated fats in food? Dietitians Association of Australia website. https://daa.asn.au/smart-eating-for-you/smart-eating-fast-facts/nourishing-nutrients/where-do-i-find-saturated-fats-in-food/. Accessed March 1, 2019.

193. Smart Balance. Palm Kernel Oil vs. Palm Fruit Oil. Smart Balance website. https://www.smartbalance.com/nutrition/topics/palmkernaloil. Accessed March 4, 2018.

194. US National Library of Medicine. Palm Oil. MedlinePlus website. https://medlineplus.gov/druginfo/natural/1139.html. Published 2018. Accessed March 4, 2019.

195. American Heart Association. Trans Fats. American Heart Association website. https://www.heart.org/en/healthy-living/healthy-eating/eat-smart/fats/trans-fat. Accessed March 2, 2019.

196. Center for Science in the Public Interest. *Artificial Trans Fat: A Timeline*. https://cspinet.org/sites/default/files/attachment/trans%20fat%20timeline.pdf. Accessed March 1, 2019.

197. Oliveira R. The Frightening Facts About Trans Fats. UC Davis Integrative Medicine website. https://ucdintegrativemedicine.com/2016/08/frightening-facts-trans-fats/#gs.i90bi34s. Published 2016. Accessed March 1, 2019.

198. Fuhrman J, Ferreri DM. Fueling the Vegetarian (Vegan) Athlete. *Curr Sports Med Rep*. 2010;9(4):233-241. doi:10.1249/JSR.0b013e3181e93a6f

199. ConsumerLab.com. Fish Oil and Omega-3 and -7 Supplements Review (Including Krill, Algal, Calamari, and Sea Buckthorn Oil Supplements). ConsumerLab.com website. https://www.consumerlab.com/reviews/fish_oil_supplements_review/omega3/. Published 2018. Accessed March 1, 2019.

200. Coconut Oil. Harvard T.H. Chan School of Public Health website. https://www.hsph.harvard.edu/nutritionsource/food-features/coconut-oil/. Accessed October 5, 2018.

201. Eyres L, Eyres MF, Chisholm A, Brown RC. Coconut oil consumption and cardiovascular risk factors in humans. *Nutr Rev*. 2016;74(4):267-280. doi:10.1093/nutrit/nuw002

202. Fabian MD. Properties of Lauric Acid and Their Significance in Coconut Oil. *J Am Oil Chem Soc*. 2015. http://agris.fao.org/agris-search/search.do?recordID=US201500145450. Accessed March 1, 2019.

203. American Heart Association. HDL (Good), LDL (Bad) Cholesterol and Triglycerides. American Heart Association website. http://www.heart.org/en/health-topics/cholesterol/hdl-good-ldl-bad-cholesterol-and-triglycerides. Accessed October 5, 2018.

204. Hultin G. Is MCT Oil a Miracle Supplement or Just Another Fad? Food & Nutrition Magazine website. https://foodandnutrition.org/january-february-2016/mct-oil-miracle-supplement-just-another-fad/. Published 2015. Accessed October 5, 2018.

205. Parrish CR. *The Use of Medium-Chain Triglycerides in Gastrointestinal Disorders*. *Practical Gastroenteroly*. *2017*. https://med.virginia.edu/ginutrition/wp-content/uploads/sites/199/2014/06/Parrish-February-17.pdf. Accessed October 5, 2018.

206. Wang Y, Liu Z, Han Y, Xu J, Huang W, Li Z. Medium Chain Triglycerides enhances exercise endurance through the increased mitochondrial biogenesis and metabolism. *PLoS One*. 2018;13(2):e0191182. doi:10.1371/journal.pone.0191182

207. ConsumerLab.com. Medium-Chain Triglycerides. Consumerlab.com website. https://www.consumerlab.com/tnp.asp?chunkiid=21809&login=success. Published 2015. Accessed March 2, 2019.

208. Judith C. Thalheimer. Coconut Oil. Today's Dietitian website. https://www.todaysdietitian.com/newarchives/1016p32.shtml. Published 2016. Accessed March 2, 2019.

209. ConsumerLab.com. Coconut Oil and Medium Chain Triglycerides (MCT Oil) Review. ConsumerLab.com website. https://www.consumerlab.com/reviews/coconut-and-MCT-oils/coconut-mct-oil/. Published 2019.

210. St-Onge MP, Bosarge A, Goree LL, Darnell B. Medium chain triglyceride oil consumption as part of a weight loss diet does not lead to an adverse metabolic profile when compared to olive oil. *J Am Coll Nutr*. 2008;27(5):547-552. http://www.ncbi.nlm.nih.gov/pubmed/18845704. Accessed October 5, 2018.

211. Clegg ME. Medium-chain triglycerides are advantageous in promoting weight loss although not beneficial to exercise performance. *Int J Food Sci Nutr*. 2010;61(7):653-679. doi:10.3109/09637481003702114

212. Pike A. Keto Diet 101: What to Know Before You Commit. The International Food Information Council (IFIC) Foundation website. https://foodinsight.org/keto-diet-101-what-to-know-before-you-commit/.

213. Ketogenic diet. Healthdirect website. https://www.healthdirect.gov.au/ketogenic-diet. Updated 2019. Accessed March 2, 2019.

214. Roehl K, Sewak SL. Practice Paper of the Academy of Nutrition and Dietetics: Classic and Modified Ketogenic Diets for Treatment of Epilepsy. *J Acad Nutr Diet.* 2017;117(8):1279-1292. doi:10.1016/j.jand.2017.06.006

215. Wroble KA, Trott MN, Schweitzer GG, Rahman RS, Kelly P V, Weiss EP. Low-carbohydrate, ketogenic diet impairs anaerobic exercise performance in exercise-trained women and men: a randomized-sequence crossover trial. *J Sports Med Phys Fitness.* April 2018. doi:10.23736/S0022-4707.18.08318-4

216. Heavey PM. Webb GP. Dietary Supplements and Functional Foods. *Br J Nutr.* 2006;96(06):1172. doi:10.1017/BJN20061886

217. National Institutes of Health Office of Dietary Supplements. Iodine Fact Sheet for Health Professionals. National Institutes of Health Office of Dietary Supplements website. https://ods.od.nih.gov/factsheets/iodine-healthprofessional/. Accessed March 3, 2019.

218. U.S. National Library of Medicine National Center for Biotechnology Information. Compound Summary- Serotonin. PubChem website. https://pubchem.ncbi.nlm.nih.gov/compound/serotonin. Accessed April 4, 2019.

219. National Institutes of Health Office of Dietary Supplements. Vitamin B12 Fact Sheet for Health Professionals. National Institutes of Health Office of Dietary Supplements website. https://ods.od.nih.gov/factsheets/VitaminB12-HealthProfessional/. Accessed September 25, 2018.

220. Rizzo G, Laganà AS, Rapisarda AMC, et al. Vitamin B12 among Vegetarians: Status, Assessment and Supplementation. *Nutrients.* 2016;8(12). doi:10.3390/nu8120767

221. Teas J, Pino S, Critchley A, Braverman LE. Variability of Iodine Content in Common Commercially Available Edible Seaweeds. *Thyroid.* 2004;14(10):836-841. doi:10.1089/thy.2004.14.836

222. Ershow AG, Skeaff SA, Merkel JM, Pehrsson PR. Development of Databases on Iodine in Foods and Dietary Supplements. *Nutrients.* 2018;10(1). doi:10.3390/nu10010100

223. National Institutes of Health Office of Dietary Supplements. Iron Fact Sheet for Consumers. National Institutes of Health Office of Dietary Supplements website. https://ods.od.nih.gov/factsheets/Iron-Consumer/. Accessed March 2, 2019.

224. Pasricha SR, Low M, Thompson J, Farrell A, De-Regil LM. Iron Supplementation Benefits Physical Performance in Women of Reproductive Age: A Systematic Review and Meta-Analysis. *J Nutr.* 2014;144(6):906-914. doi:10.3945/jn.113.189589

225. Wouthuyzen-Bakker M, van Assen S. Exercise-induced anaemia: a forgotten cause of iron deficiency anaemia in young adults. *Br J Gen Pract.* 2015;65(634):268-269. doi:10.3399/bjgp15X685069

226. Sports Dietitians Australia. Fact Sheet - *Iron Depletion in Athletes What Does Iron Do in the Body?* https://www.sportsdietitians.com.au/wp-content/uploads/2015/04/Iron_depletion_in_athletes.pdf. Accessed March 2, 2019.

227. Brumitt J, McIntosh L, Rutt R. Comprehensive Sports Medicine Treatment of an Athlete Who Runs Cross-Country and is Iron Deficient. *N Am J Sports Phys Ther.* 2009;4(1):13-20. http://www.ncbi.nlm.nih.gov/pubmed/21509116. Accessed March 2, 2019.

228. National Institutes of Health Office of Dietary Supplements. Iron Fact Sheet for Health Professionals. National Institutes of Health Office of Dietary Supplements website. https://ods.od.nih.gov/factsheets/Iron-HealthProfessional/. Accessed April 4, 2019.

229. US National Library of Medicine. Iron in diet. MedlinePlus website. https://medlineplus.gov/ency/article/002422.htm. Accessed March 2, 2019.

230. Basuli D, Stevens RG, Torti FM, Torti S V. Epidemiological associations between iron and cardiovascular disease and diabetes. *Front Pharmacol.* 2014;5:117. doi:10.3389/fphar.2014.00117

231. Brittin HC, Nossaman CE. Iron content of food cooked in iron utensils. *J Am Diet Assoc.* 1986;86(7):897-901. http://www.ncbi.nlm.nih.gov/pubmed/3722654. Accessed March 15, 2019.

232. Statuta SM, Asif IM, Drezner JA. Relative energy deficiency in sport (RED-S). *Br J Sports Med.* 2017;51(21):1570-1571. doi:10.1136/bjsports-2017-097700

233. Chu A, Petocz P, Samman S. Immediate Effects of Aerobic Exercise on Plasma/Serum Zinc Levels. *Med Sci Sport Exerc.* 2016;48(4):726-733. doi:10.1249/MSS.0000000000000805

234. National Institutes of Health Office of Dietary Supplements. Zinc Fact Sheet for Health Professionals. National Institutes of Health Office of Dietary Supplements website. https://ods.od.nih.gov/factsheets/Zinc-HealthProfessional/. Accessed March 2, 2019.

235. Simopoulos AP. Omega-3 fatty acids and athletics. *Curr Sports Med Rep.* 2007;6(4):230-236. http://www.ncbi.nlm.nih.gov/pubmed/17617998. Accessed March 2, 2019.

236. Philpott JD, Witard OC, Galloway SDR. Applications of omega-3 polyunsaturated fatty acid supplementation for sport performance. *Res Sport Med.* November 2018:1-19. doi:10.1080/15438627.2018.1550401

237. Smith GI, Atherton P, Reeds DN, et al. Omega-3 polyunsaturated fatty acids augment the muscle protein anabolic response to hyperinsulinaemia-hyperaminoacidaemia in healthy young and middle-aged men and women. *Clin Sci (Lond)*. 2011;121(6):267-278. doi:10.1042/CS20100597

238. Smith GI, Atherton P, Reeds DN, et al. Dietary omega-3 fatty acid supplementation increases the rate of muscle protein synthesis in older adults: a randomized controlled trial. *Am J Clin Nutr*. 2011;93(2):402-412. doi:10.3945/ajcn.110.005611

239. Campbell T. A plant-based diet and stroke. *J Geriatr Cardiol*. 2017;14(5):321-326. doi:10.11909/j.issn.1671-5411.2017.05.010

240. U.S. Department of Health and Human Services and U.S. Department of Agriculture. Chapter 1: Key Recommendations: Components of Healthy Eating Patterns - 2015-2020 Dietary Guidelines. https://health.gov/dietaryguidelines/2015/guidelines/chapter-1/key-recommendations/. Accessed April 4, 2019.

241. National Heart, Lung, and Blood Institute. DASH Eating Plan. National Heart, Lung, and Blood Institute website. https://www.nia.nih.gov/health/dash-eating-plan. Accessed March 2, 2019.

242. Morris MC, Tangney CC, Wang Y, et al. MIND diet slows cognitive decline with aging. *Alzheimers Dement*. 2015;11(9):1015-1022. doi:10.1016/j.jalz.2015.04.011

243. Pike A. What is the Nordic Diet? International Food Information Council Foundation website. https://foodinsight.org/what-is-the-nordic-diet/. Published 2018.

244. American Institute for Cancer Research. Alcohol and cancer risk. American Institute for Cancer Research (AICR) website. http://www.aicr.org/reduce-your-cancer-risk/diet/alcohol-and-cancer-risk.html. Accessed March 3, 2019.

245. U.S. Department of Health and Human Services and U.S. Department of Agriculture. Appendix 9. Alcohol. Dietary Guidelines 2015-2020. https://health.gov/dietaryguidelines/2015/guidelines/appendix-9/. Accessed March 15, 2019.

246. United States Olympic Committee. Nutrition. United States Olympic Committee website. https://www.teamusa.org/nutrition. Accessed March 1, 2019.

247. Liu RH. Whole grain phytochemicals and health. *J Cereal Sci*. 2007;46(3):207-219. doi:10.1016/j.jcs.2007.06.010

248. Webb D. Phytochemicals' Role in Good Health. Today's Dietitian website. https://www.todaysdietitian.com/newarchives/090313p70.shtml. Published 2013. Accessed October 2, 2018.

249. Coco MG, Vinson JA, Vinson JA. Analysis of Popcorn (Zea mays L. var. everta) for Antioxidant Capacity and Total Phenolic Content. *Antioxidants (Basel, Switzerland)*. 2019;8(1). doi:10.3390/antiox8010022

250. Poulose SM, Miller MG, Shukitt-Hale B. Role of Walnuts in Maintaining Brain Health with Age. *J Nutr.* 2014;144(4):561S-566S. doi:10.3945/jn.113.184838

251. Wang J, Song Y, Chen Z, Leng SX. Connection between Systemic Inflammation and Neuroinflammation Underlies Neuroprotective Mechanism of Several Phytochemicals in Neurodegenerative Diseases. *Oxid Med Cell Longev.* 2018;2018:1-16. doi:10.1155/2018/1972714

252. Zhang YJ, Gan RY, Li S, et al. Antioxidant Phytochemicals for the Prevention and Treatment of Chronic Diseases. *Molecules.* 2015;20(12):21138-21156. doi:10.3390/molecules201219753

253. Bhagwat S, Haytowitz DB, Holden JM. *USDA Database for the Flavonoid Content of Selected Foods Release 3.1.* 2013. https://www.ars.usda.gov/ARSUserFiles/80400525/Data/Flav/Flav_R03-1.pdf. Accessed March 15, 2019.

254. Barbieri R, Coppo E, Marchese A, et al. Phytochemicals for human disease: An update on plant-derived compounds antibacterial activity. *Microbiol Res.* 2017;196:44-68. doi:10.1016/J.MICRES.2016.12.003

255. Kuršvietienė L, Stanevičienė I, Mongirdienė A, Bernatonienė J. Multiplicity of effects and health benefits of resveratrol. *Elsevier.* 2016;52(3):148-55. doi: 10.1016/j.medici.2016.03.003

256. Li Y, Yao J, Han C, et al. Quercetin, Inflammation and Immunity. *Nutrients.* 2016;8(3):167. doi:10.3390/nu8030167

257. Dull A-M, Moga MA, Dimienescu OG, et al. Therapeutic Approaches of Resveratrol on Endometriosis via Anti-Inflammatory and Anti-Angiogenic Pathways. *Molecules.* 2019;24(4):667. doi:10.3390/molecules24040667

258. Chandrasekara A, Josheph Kumar T. Roots and Tuber Crops as Functional Foods: A Review on Phytochemical Constituents and Their Potential Health Benefits. *Int J Food Sci.* 2016;2016:1-15. doi:10.1155/2016/3631647

259. Goncharov N, Orekhov AN, Voitenko N, Ukolov A, Jenkins R, Avdonin P. Organosulfur Compounds as Nutraceuticals. *Nutraceuticals.* January 2016:555-568. doi:10.1016/B978-0-12-802147-7.00041-3

260. Halvorsen BL, Carlsen MH, Phillips KM, et al. Content of redox-active compounds (ie, antioxidants) in foods consumed in the United States. *Am J Clin Nutr.* 2006;84(1):95-135. doi:10.1093/ajcn/84.1.95

261. Henning SM, Zhang Y, Seeram NP, et al. Antioxidant capacity and phytochemical content of herbs and spices in dry, fresh and blended herb paste form. *Int J Food Sci Nutr.* 2011;62(3):219-225. doi:10.3109/09637486.2010.530595

262. Ederle S. Did You Know... Veggies' unique colors are packed with health promoting power? SuperKids Nutrition website. http://www.superkidsnutrition.com/ fv_vegetable-color/. Accessed October 2, 2018.

263. American Optometric Association. Lutein and Zeaxanthin - Eye-Friendly Nutrients. American Optometric Association website. https://www.aoa.org/patients-and-public/caring-for-your-vision/nutrition/lutein-and-zeaxanthin. Accessed October 2, 2018.

264. Simonne AH, Smith M, Weaver DB, Vail T, Barnes S, Wei CI. Retention and changes of soy isoflavones and carotenoids in immature soybean seeds (Edamame) during processing. *J Agric Food Chem*. 2000;48(12):6061-6069. http://www.ncbi.nlm.nih.gov/ pubmed/11141271. Accessed October 2, 2018.

265. Henneman A. See RED on Valentine's Day. Institute of Agriculture and Natural Resources University of Nebraska-Lincoln website. https://food.unl.edu/see-red-valentines-day. Accessed October 2, 2018.

266. Carotenoids -Carotene, -Carotene, -Cryptoxanthin, Lycopene, Lutein, and Zeaxanthin. Linus Pauling Institute Oregon State University website. https://lpi.oregon-state.edu/mic/dietary-factors/phytochemicals/carotenoids. Accessed October 2, 2018.

267. Stanford Cancer Nutrition Services. *Phytochemicals: The Cancer Fighters in the Foods We Eat*. Stanford Healthcare website. https://stanfordhealthcare.org/content/ dam/SHC/programs-services/cancer-nutrition/docs/phytochemicals-during-cancer-treatment-nutrition-facts.pdf. Accessed October 2, 2018.

268. Mbagwu F., Okafor VU, Ekeanyanwu J. Phytochemical screening on four edible legumes (Vigna subterranean, Glycine max, Arachis hypogea, and Vigna uniguiculata) found in eastern Nigeria. *African J Plant Sci*. 2011;5(6):370-372. Accessed October 2, 2018.

269. Soy Isoflavones | Linus Pauling Institute Oregon State University website. https:// lpi.oregonstate.edu/mic/dietary-factors/phytochemicals/soy-isoflavones. Accessed October 2, 2018.

270. Pérez-Jiménez J, Neveu V, Vos F, Scalbert A. Identification of the 100 richest dietary sources of polyphenols: an application of the Phenol-Explorer database. *Eur J Clin Nutr*. 2010;64(S3):S112-S120. doi:10.1038/ejcn.2010.221

271. American Institute for Cancer Research. The Cancer Fighters in Your Food. https://store.aicr.org/products/the-cancer-fighters-in-your-food. Accessed October 2, 2018.

272. Mlcek J, Jurikova T, Skrovankova S, Sochor J. Quercetin and Its Anti-Allergic Immune Response. *Molecules*. 2016;21(5):623. doi:10.3390/molecules21050623

273. Center for Disease Control and Prevention. *2018 State Indicator Report on Fruits and Vegetables.* https://www.cdc.gov/nutrition/downloads/fruits-vegetables/2018/2018-fruit-vegetable-report-508.pdf. Accessed April 4, 2019.

274. Brown AC. *Understanding Food: Principles and Preparation.* Boston, MA: Cengage; 2018.

275. Guiden K. Going Cuckoo for Cacao. International Federation of Food Insight Foundation website. https://foodinsight.org/going-cuckoo-for-cacao/. Accessed March 3, 2019.

276. Di Mattia CD, Sacchetti G, Mastrocola D, Serafini M. From Cocoa to Chocolate: The Impact of Processing on In Vitro Antioxidant Activity and the Effects of Chocolate on Antioxidant Markers In Vivo. *Front Immunol.* 2017;8:1207. doi:10.3389/fimmu.2017.01207

277. Thomas DT, Erdman KA, Burke LM. Position of the Academy of Nutrition and Dietetics, Dietitians of Canada, and the American College of Sports Medicine: Nutrition and Athletic Performance. *J Acad Nutr Diet.* 2016;116(3):501-528. doi:10.1016/j.jand.2015.12.006

278. National Institutes of Health Office of Dietary Supplements. Dietary Supplements for Exercise and Athletic Performance Fact Sheet for Consumers. National Institutes of Health Office of Dietary Supplements website. https://ods.od.nih.gov/factsheets/ExerciseAndAthleticPerformance-Consumer/. Accessed March 2, 2019.

279. US Food & Drug Administration. What You Need to Know About Dietary Supplements. US Food & Drug Administration website. https://www.fda.gov/Food/Dietary-Supplements/UsingDietarySupplements/ucm109760.htm. Accessed March 2, 2019.

280. Statement from FDA Commissioner Scott Gottlieb, M.D., on the agency's new efforts to strengthen regulation of dietary supplements by modernizing and reforming FDA's oversight. https://www.fda.gov/NewsEvents/Newsroom/PressAnnouncements/ucm631065.htm. Accessed March 15, 2019.

281. Almendarez S. The End of Proprietary Blends and other Supplement Issues for Sports Dietitians. Natural Products Insider website. https://www.naturalproductsinsider.com/sports-nutrition/end-proprietary-blends-and-other-supplement-issues-sports-dietitians. Published 2014. Accessed March 2, 2019.

282. Franek F, Hohenwarter O, Katinger H. Plant Protein Hydrolysates: Preparation of Defined Peptide Fractions Promoting Growth and Production in Animal Cells Cultures. *Biotechnol Prog.* 2000;16(5):688-692. doi:10.1021/bp0001011

283. Clean Label Project. Protein Powder. Clean Label Project website. https://www.cleanlabelproject.org/protein-powder/. Accessed March 15, 2019.

284. ConsumerLabs.com. *Product Review: Protein Powders, Shakes, and Drinks Review*. ConsumerLabs.com website. https://www.consumerlab.com/reviews/Protein_Powders_Shakes_Drinks_Sports/NutritionDrinks/. Published 2018.

285. NSF International Certified for Sport®. NSF International Certified for Sport website. http://www.nsfsport.com/. Accessed April 4, 2019.

286. Informed-Sport Trusted by sport. Informed-Sport website. https://www.informed-sport.com/. Accessed April 4, 2019.

287. Informed-Choice Trusted by Sport. Informed-Choice website. https://www.informed-choice.org/. Accessed April 4, 2019.

288. U.S. Pharmacopeia. http://www.usp.org/. Accessed April 4, 2019.

289. Holwerda AM, Overkamp M, Paulussen KJM, et al. Protein Supplementation after Exercise and before Sleep Does Not Further Augment Muscle Mass and Strength Gains during Resistance Exercise Training in Active Older Men. *J Nutr*. 2018;148(11):1723-1732. doi:10.1093/jn/nxy169

290. Hashimoto R, Sakai A, Murayama M, et al. Effects of dietary soy protein on skeletal muscle volume and strength in humans with various physical activities. *J Med Investig*. 2015;62(3.4):177-183. doi:10.2152/jmi.62.177

291. Hulmi JJ, Lockwood CM, Stout JR. Effect of protein/essential amino acids and resistance training on skeletal muscle hypertrophy: A case for whey protein. *Nutr Metab (Lond)*. 2010;7(1):51. doi:10.1186/1743-7075-7-51

292. Sports Dietitians of Australia. Protein Supplementation. Sports Dietitians Australia (SDA) website. https://www.sportsdietitians.com.au/factsheets/supplements/protein-supplementation/. Accessed March 2, 2019.

293. Micellar Casein Protein Powder 5lb - Naked Casein. Naked Nutrition website. https://nkdnutrition.com/products/micellar-casein-protein-powder. Accessed March 3, 2019.

294. Egg White Protein Powder - 3lb GMO Free. Naked Nutrition website. https://nkdnutrition.com/products/egg-white-protein-powder. Accessed March 3, 2019.

295. Lugo JP, Saiyed ZM, Lau FC, et al. Undenatured type II collagen (UC-II®) for joint support: a randomized, double-blind, placebo-controlled study in healthy volunteers. *J Int Soc Sports Nutr*. 2013;10(1):48. doi:10.1186/1550-2783-10-48

296. Crowley DC, Lau FC, Sharma P, et al. Safety and efficacy of undenatured type II collagen in the treatment of osteoarthritis of the knee: a clinical trial. *Int J Med Sci*. 2009;6(6):312-321. http://www.ncbi.nlm.nih.gov/pubmed/19847319. Accessed March 15, 2019.

---

297. Monro JA, Leon R, Puri BK. The risk of lead contamination in bone broth diets. *Med Hypotheses*. 2013;80(4):389-390. doi:10.1016/j.mehy.2012.12.026

298. Silvipriya K, Kumar K, Bhat A, Kumar B, John A, Lakshmanan P. Collagen: Animal Sources and Biomedical Application. *J Appl Pharm Sci*. 2015;123-127. doi:10.7324/JAPS.2015.50322

299. Clark KL, Sebastianelli W, Flechsenhar KR, et al. 24-Week study on the use of collagen hydrolysate as a dietary supplement in athletes with activity-related joint pain. *Curr Med Res Opin*. 2008;24(5):1485-1496. doi:10.1185/030079908X291967

300. Bruyère O, Zegels B, Leonori L, et al. Effect of collagen hydrolysate in articular pain: A 6-month randomized, double-blind, placebo controlled study. *Complement Ther Med*. 2012;20(3):124-130. doi:10.1016/j.ctim.2011.12.007

301. Schunck M, Zague V, Oesser S, Proksch E. Dietary Supplementation with Specific Collagen Peptides Has a Body Mass Index-Dependent Beneficial Effect on Cellulite Morphology. *J Med Food*. 2015;18(12):1340-1348. doi:10.1089/jmf.2015.0022

302. Proksch E, Schunck M, Zague V, Segger D, Degwert J, Oesser S. Oral Intake of Specific Bioactive Collagen Peptides Reduces Skin Wrinkles and Increases Dermal Matrix Synthesis. *Skin Pharmacol Physiol*. 2014;27(3):113-119. doi:10.1159/000355523

303. Levine M, Violet PC. Breaking down, starting up: can a vitamin C–enriched gelatin supplement before exercise increase collagen synthesis? *Am J Clin Nutr*. 2017;105(1):5-7. doi:10.3945/ajcn.116.148312

304. Shaw G, Lee-Barthel A, Ross ML, Wang B, Baar K. Vitamin C–enriched gelatin supplementation before intermittent activity augments collagen synthesis. *Am J Clin Nutr*. 2017;105(1):136-143. doi:10.3945/ajcn.116.138594

305. Dressler P, Gehring D, Zdzieblik D, Oesser S, Gollhofer A, König D. Improvement of Functional Ankle Properties Following Supplementation with Specific Collagen Peptides in Athletes with Chronic Ankle Instability. *J Sports Sci Med*. 2018;17(2):298-304. http://www.ncbi.nlm.nih.gov/pubmed/29769831. Accessed March 2, 2019.

306. Hays NP, Kim H, Wells AM, Kajkenova O, Evans WJ. Effects of Whey and Fortified Collagen Hydrolysate Protein Supplements on Nitrogen Balance and Body Composition in Older Women. *J Am Diet Assoc*. 2009;109(6):1082-1087. doi:10.1016/j.jada.2009.03.003

307. Zdzieblik D, Oesser S, Baumstark MW, Gollhofer A, König D. Collagen peptide supplementation in combination with resistance training improves body composition and increases muscle strength in elderly sarcopenic men: a randomised controlled trial. *Br J Nutr*. 2015;114(8):1237-1245. doi:10.1017/S0007114515002810

308. Gorissen SHM, Crombag JJR, Senden JMG, et al. Protein content and amino acid composition of commercially available plant-based protein isolates. *Amino Acids.* 2018;50(12):1685-1695. doi:10.1007/s00726-018-2640-5

309. Babault N, Païzis C, Deley G, et al. Pea proteins oral supplementation promotes muscle thickness gains during resistance training: a double-blind, randomized, Placebo-controlled clinical trial vs. Whey protein. *J Int Soc Sports Nutr.* 2015;12(1):3. doi:10.1186/s12970-014-0064-5

310. Pea Protein Powder 5lb - Vegan & Gluten Free - Naked Pea. Naked Nutrition website. https://nkdnutrition.com/products/pea-protein-powder. Accessed March 3, 2019.

311. Messina M, Lynch H, Dickinson JM, Reed KE. No Difference Between the Effects of Supplementing With Soy Protein Versus Animal Protein on Gains in Muscle Mass and Strength in Response to Resistance Exercise. *Int J Sport Nutr Exerc Metab.* 2018;28(6):674-685. doi:10.1123/ijsnem.2018-0071

312. Hartman JW, Tang JE, Wilkinson SB, et al. Consumption of fat-free fluid milk after resistance exercise promotes greater lean mass accretion than does consumption of soy or carbohydrate in young, novice, male weightlifters. *Am J Clin Nutr.* 2007;86(2):373-381. doi:10.1093/ajcn/86.2.373

313. Joy JM, Lowery RP, Wilson JM, et al. The effects of 8 weeks of whey or rice protein supplementation on body composition and exercise performance. *Nutr J.* 2013;12(1):86. doi:10.1186/1475-2891-12-86

314. Organic Brown Rice Protein Powder - Naked Rice - 5lb. Naked Nutrition website. https://nkdnutrition.com/products/organic-brown-rice-protein-powder. Accessed March 3, 2019.

315. *Sport, Cardiovascular, and Wellness Dietitians. Caffeine and Athletic Performance.* http://www.sportsrd.org/wp-content/uploads/2018/11/Caffeine_and_Athletic_Performance_WEB.pdf. Accessed March 29, 2019.

316. Starbucks. *Beverage Nutrition Information.* https://globalassets.starbucks.com/assets/94fbcc2ab1e24359850fa1870fc988bc.pdf. Accessed April 4, 2019.

317. Starbucks. Cold Brew Coffee. Starbucks website. https://www.starbucks.com/menu/drinks/brewed-coffee/cold-brew-coffee. Accessed April 4, 2019.

318. How to use 5-hour ENERGY® Shots. 5-hour Energy website. https://5hourenergy.com/facts/how-to-use/. Accessed April 4, 2019.

319. Kreider RB, Kalman DS, Antonio J, et al. International Society of Sports Nutrition position stand: safety and efficacy of creatine supplementation in exercise, sport, and medicine. *J Int Soc Sports Nutr.* 2017;14:18. doi:10.1186/s12970-017-0173-z

320. ConsumerLab.com. Product Reviews, Muscle & Workout Supplements Review (Creatine and Branched-chain Amino Acids). ConsumerLab.com website. https://www.consumerlab.com/reviews/review_creatine_BCAAs/creatine/.

321. Perry D, Ketterly J. Creatine Supplementation and Athletic Performance. Sports, Cardiovascular, and Wellness Nutrition (SCAN). 2017.

322. Williams M, Kreider R, Branch D. *Nutrition for Health, Fitness and Sport*. New York, NY: McGraw-Hill Education; 2017. https://www.researchgate.net/figure/Creatine-Content-in-Select-Foods_tbl3_227249571. Accessed April 4, 2019.

323. US National Library of Medicine. Guarana. MedlinePlus website. https://medlineplus.gov/druginfo/natural/935.html. Published 2018.

324. US National Library of Medicine. Yerba Mate: MedlinePlus Supplements. MedlinePlus website. https://medlineplus.gov/druginfo/natural/828.html#Safety. Published 2018. Accessed March 29, 2019.

325. National Institutes of Health Office of Dietary Supplements. Dietary Supplements for Weight Loss Fact Sheet for Health Professionals. https://ods.od.nih.gov/factsheets/WeightLoss-HealthProfessional/. Accessed March 29, 2019.

326. Campbell B, Wilborn C, La Bounty P, et al. International Society of Sports Nutrition position stand: energy drinks. *J Int Soc Sports Nutr*. 2013;10(1):1. doi:10.1186/1550-2783-10-1

327. ConsumerLab.com - independent tests and reviews of vitamin, mineral, and herbal supplements. Consumerlab.com website. https://www.consumerlab.com/. Accessed March 29, 2019.

328. National Institute of Health Office of Dietary Supplements. Dietary Supplements for Exercise and Athletic Performance Fact Sheet for Health Professionals. https://ods.od.nih.gov/factsheets/ExerciseAndAthleticPerformance-HealthProfessional/. Updated June 2017.

329. Nutrition Care Manual. https://www.nutritioncaremanual.org/?err=NLI. Accessed March 29, 2019.

330. Naik SD, Freudenberger RS. Ephedra–Associated Cardiomyopathy. *Ann Pharmacother*. 2004;38(3):400-403. doi:10.1345/aph.1D408

331. National Collegiate Athletic Association. 2018-19 NCAA Banned Drugs List. NCAA website. http://www.ncaa.org/2018-19-ncaa-banned-drugs-list. Accessed March 29, 2019.

332. Sports Dietitians Australia (SDA). Nitrate (Beetroot Juice). Sports Dietitians Australia website. https://www.sportsdietitians.com.au/factsheets/supplements/beetroot-juice-nitrate/. Accessed March 2, 2019.

333. Chhikara N, Kushwaha K, Sharma P, Gat Y, Panghal A. Bioactive compounds of beetroot and utilization in food processing industry: A critical review. *Food Chem.* 2019;272:192-200. doi:10.1016/J.FOODCHEM.2018.08.022

334. Lidder S, Webb AJ. Vascular effects of dietary nitrate (as found in green leafy vegetables and beetroot) via the nitrate-nitrite-nitric oxide pathway. *Br J Clin Pharmacol.* 2013;75(3):677-696. doi:10.1111/j.1365-2125.2012.04420.x

335. Shehzad A, Qureshi M, Anwar MN, Lee YS. Multifunctional Curcumin Mediate Multitherapeutic Effects. *J Food Sci.* 2017;82(9):2006-2015. doi: 10.1111/1750-3841.13793

336. Kuptniratsaikul V, Thanakhumtorn S, Chinswangwatanakul P, Wattanamongkonsil L, Thamlikitkul V. Efficacy and Safety of Curcuma domestica Extracts in Patients with Knee Osteoarthritis. *J Altern Complement Med.* 2009;15(8):891-897. doi:10.1089/acm.2008.0186

337. Taylor K. Fruits and Vegetables: Nature's Cancer Prevention. Iowa State University Extension and Outreach website. https://blogs.extension.iastate.edu/wellness/2013/07/30/fruits-and-vegetables-natures-cancer-prevention/. Accessed March 15, 2019.

338. Drobnic F, Riera J, Appendino G, et al. Reduction of delayed onset muscle soreness by a novel curcumin delivery system (Meriva®): a randomised, placebo-controlled trial. *J Int Soc Sports Nutr.* 2014;11(1):31. doi:10.1186/1550-2783-11-31

339. United States Department of Agriculture Agricultural Research Service. Basic Report: 02043, Spices, turmeric, ground. USDA Food Composition Databases website. https://ndb.nal.usda.gov/ndb/foods/show?ndbno=02043. Accessed March 2, 2019.

340. United States Department of Agriculture Agricultural Research Service. Spices, parsley, dried. USDA Food Composition Databases website. https://ndb.nal.usda.gov/ndb/foods/show/299569. Accessed March 15, 2019.

341. United States Department of Agriculture Agricultural Research Service. Basic Report: 02029, Spices, bay leaf. USDA Food Composition Databases website. https://ndb.nal.usda.gov/ndb/foods/show/254. Accessed March 15, 2019.

342. National Center for Complimentary and Integrative Health. Garlic. National Center for Complimentary and Integrative Health website. https://nccih.nih.gov/health/garlic/ataglance.htm. Accessed March 15, 2019.

343. Garlic - Garlic and Organosulfur Compounds. Linus Pauling Institute Oregon State University website. https://lpi.oregonstate.edu/mic/food-beverages/garlic. Accessed March 15, 2019.

Index

C

W

Z

Made in the USA
Monee, IL
10 December 2019